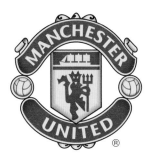

MANCHESTER UNITED
OFFICIAL YEARBOOK 2002

Compiled and Edited by Cliff Butler
Assisted by Ivan Ponting

Contributors
MARTIN EDWARDS
SIR ALEX FERGUSON
BARRY MOORHOUSE
CLIFF BUTLER
IVAN PONTING

Thanks to
ARTHUR ALBISTON, NEIL BAILEY, JULIAN BARKER, ADAM BOSTOCK, STEVE BOWER, PHIL BROGAN, DAVE BUSHELL, DIANE CLIFFORD, JOHN COOKE, TONY COTON, MIKE COX, RACHEL CROSS, JIMMY CURRAN, PAUL DAVIES, SIMON DAVIES, MARK DEMPSEY, MARK EDWARDS, SHARON FAULKNER, BRIAN FINCH, JULIAN FLANDERS, LES KERSHAW, TREVOR LEA, EDDIE LEACH, MARK LLOYD, BRIAN McCLAIR, PAUL MCGUINNESS, TOMMY MARTIN, STUART MATHIESON, DAVID MEEK, ROSS MILLARD, ALBERT MORGAN, DEREK NASSARI, CLARE NICHOLAS, TOMMY O'NEIL, MIKE PHELAN, MICK PRIEST, MATT PROCTOR, DAVID PUGH, KEN RAMSDEN, MARIE RILEY, ARTHUR ROBERTS, DAVE ROUSE, DAVID RYAN, JIMMY RYAN, JIM SANDFORD, ANDY SMITH, TOM STATHAM, CRAIG STEVENS, REBECCA TOW, TONY WHELAN, DAVID WILLIAMS, KATHIE WILSON, NEIL WITHERS, STUART WORTHINGTON, ALEC WYLIE, ANNE WYLIE AND EVERYONE WHO SUPPLIED INFORMATION THROUGHOUT THE 2001-2002 SEASON.

THANKS ALSO TO ALL THE CLUBS WHO KINDLY GRANTED PERMISSION IN ALLOWING THEIR OFFICIAL CLUB CRESTS TO BE REPRODUCED IN THIS PUBLICATION.

Photographs
JOHN AND MATTHEW PETERS/MANCHESTER UNITED FC
Design and editorial
DESIGNSECTION FROME

First published in 2002
10 9 8 7 6 5 4 3 2 1

Manufactured and distributed by
Carlton Books Limited
20 Mortimer Street
London W1T 3JW

ISBN
0-233-05016-7

Printed and bound in the UK by
BUTLER & TANNER LTD. FROME AND LONDON

Contents

MANCHESTER UNITED
FOOTBALL CLUB PLC

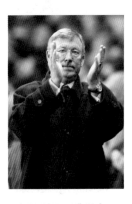

Directors	Chief Executive
C.M. EDWARDS (Chairman)	P.F. KENYON
J.M. EDELSON	
SIR BOBBY CHARLTON CBE	Manager
E.M. WATKINS LI.M.	SIR ALEX FERGUSON CBE
R.L. OLIVE	Secretary
P.F. KENYON	KENNETH R. MERRETT
D.A. GILL	

Honours

EUROPEAN CHAMPION CLUBS' CUP – Winners: 1968 · 1999

EUROPEAN CUP WINNERS' CUP – Winners: 1991

FA PREMIER LEAGUE – Champions: 1993 · 1994 · 1996 · 1997 · 1999 · 2000 · 2001

FOOTBALL LEAGUE DIVISION ONE – Champions: 1908 · 1911 · 1952 · 1956 · 1957 · 1965 · 1967

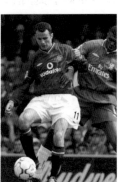

FA CHALLENGE CUP – Winners: 1909 · 1948 · 1963 · 1977 · 1983 · 1985 · 1990 · 1994 · 1996 · 1999

FOOTBALL LEAGUE CUP – Winners: 1992

INTER-CONTINENTAL CUP – Winners: 1999

UEFA SUPER CUP – Winners: 1991

FA CHARITY SHIELD – Winners: 1908 · 1911 · 1952 · 1956 · 1957 · 1983 · 1993 · 1994 · 1996 · 1997
Joint Holders: 1965 · 1967 · 1977 · 1990

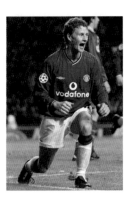

CLUB TELEPHONE NUMBERS	
Main Switchboard	0161-868 8000
Textphone for Deaf/Impaired Hearing	0161-868 8668
Ticket & Match Information	0870 757 1968
Ticket Sales	0870 442 1999
Commercial & Hospitality Sales	0870 442 1994
Megastore	0161-868 8220
Mail Order Hotline	0870 162 0212
United Review Subscriptions	0870 602 6000
Magazine Subscriptions	01458 271132
Development Association	0161-868 8600
Membership & Supporters' Club	0870 442 1994
Conference & Catering	0161-868 8450
Museum & Tour Centre	0870 442 1994
United in the Community	0161-708 9451
Manchester United Radio	0161-868 8888
Red Café	0161-868 8303
Park & Ride	0870 442 1994
Website	www.ManUtd.com
MUTV	0870 848 6888

CHAIRMAN'S MESSAGE

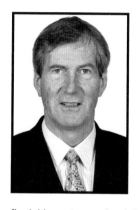

There may not have been any silverware to show for the team's efforts at the close of the season, but I don't think anyone could have any complaints about the excitement and entertainment that came our way during the campaign. We went agonisingly close on two fronts and with an ounce of luck the finale to the season could easily have ended on a happier note for us.

Reaching the last-four of the UEFA Champions League is in itself no mean feat, but that is little consolation when the final is so tantalisingly close. There is no doubt that playing against Real Madrid in the final in Glasgow, would have been an occasion to savour – particularly for Sir Alex – but ultimately we had to concede defeat to Bayer Leverkusen over two legs in the semi-final. I have to say that I thought that Bayer did extremely well in the final against Real and were unlucky not to end up with the winners' medals. The Hampden Park contest was a grand occasion which we will endeavour to emulate at the end of next season when the UEFA Champions League final will be staged at Old Trafford. That promises to be an event not to be missed, and one which will be even better if Manchester United are involved.

We were also close to claiming the Premiership for the fourth successive year, but left ourselves a little too much to do following a poor series of results in the first half of the season. The team did wonderfully well to restore themselves and take part in the title race right up until the final couple of matches. It has to be noted that it wasn't all disappointment at the end of the season. Our reserves, coached by Brian McClair, won the FA Premier Reserve League (North) for the first time whilst Neil Bailey's Under-17 side reached the final of their section where they ultimately lost out on aggregate to Newcastle United. And, the Under-19s, guided by David Williams, narrowly missed out on league honours finishing runners-up to Liverpool in their section. Congratulations to them all.

All in all it was another season of great football, high drama and wonderful entertainment. And you can re-live all the highs and lows in this the latest *Manchester United Official Yearbook*. This is the 16th year of publication and it remains an indispensable point of reference for not only United supporters, but also the press, broadcasters, students and historians of the game, and always finds a place on my bookshelf.

C. Martin Edwards

Manager's Message

I cannot deny that the thought of leading Manchester United out for the UEFA Champions League final at Hampden Park was a very exciting proposition. The famous Glasgow stadium holds many memories for me stretching back to my childhood in the city and it would indeed have been something very special to be involved in such a huge occasion just a few short miles from where I was born and brought up. I did have the odd fleeting daydream about that happening but at the same time kept telling myself that it would be a fabulous achievement if we succeeded in making it to the final.

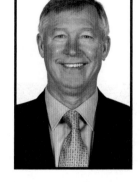

My belief in the team's capabilities of reaching the final for the second time in four seasons never faltered and even when the shattering injuries to Roy Keane and David Beckham dealt us a grievous blow I remained confident that we were more than ably equipped to overcome Bayer Leverkusen. Not for one minute did I underestimate the German team but I thought that we were in the right frame of mind to make the big step to Glasgow. Alas, it wasn't to be and while I was disappointed personally that the chance to win the European Cup in my native city had passed, the fact that we as a club had failed narrowly to reach our goal was even more distressing.

I have been in football long enough to accept that defeat is as much part of the game as winning, but losing is still hard to bear and to also relinquish our Premiership crown so close to the end of the season made it a doubly harrowing experience. I have to say that where the Premiership is concerned I thought we did really well to fight our way back into contention after that spell of games before Christmas where nothing seemed to go right. It was a terrible run of results and that we were able to pull ourselves round to give Arsenal such a good run for their money speaks volumes for the fortitude and character of our players. It was extremely disappointing not to finish the season without a trophy on the sideboard, but we can console ourselves in the knowledge that we weren't that far off the pace. It is all history now and whilst we congratulate Arsenal on winning the cup and league double, and Real Madrid on lifting the European Cup, as a club we must look forward to the fresh challenges that await us in the future.

Sir Alex Ferguson

AUGUST

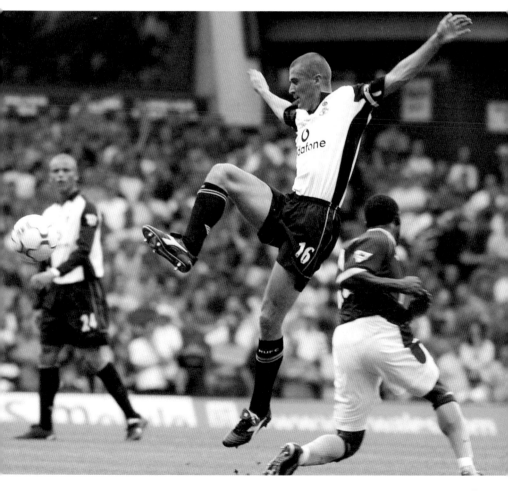

MANCHESTER UNITED 3

1. Fabien BARTHEZ
2. Gary NEVILLE
3. Denis IRWIN
4. Juan Sebastian VERON
27. Mikael SILVESTRE
6. Jaap STAM
7. David BECKHAM
18. Paul SCHOLES
12. Phil NEVILLE
10. Ruud VAN NISTELROOY
11. Ryan GIGGS

SUBSTITUTES

9. Andy COLE (12) 35
13. Roy CARROLL
15. Luke CHADWICK (10) 76
20. Ole Gunnar SOLSKJAER
24. Wesley BROWN (4) 80

BECKHAM 36
VAN NISTELROOY 51, 53

MATCH REPORT

The Red Devils made a victorious start to the latest defence of their Premiership crown, but they were matched in every department by an enterprising Fulham side which might have returned to London with all three points. True, United attacked with flair and fervour at times, with Scholes, Giggs and Beckham all prominent, and they showed characteristic grit in twice coming from behind. Another plus was the opportunism of two-goal van Nistelrooy, which whispered seductively of likely delights to come. Against that, however, the Reds were horribly and repeatedly fragile at the back, moving sluggishly to counter the pacy and inventive Cottagers, who fashioned no fewer than seven clear-cut scoring opportunities.

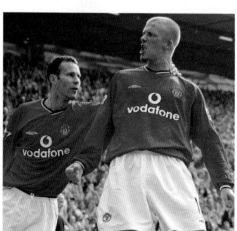

Jean Tigana's slick passers took the lead with a beautiful goal, Saha outpacing Neville before controlling a Davis through-ball with one stunning touch, then lobbing Barthez with another. The French marksman might have doubled his tally soon after, but shot wildly, then Beckham retaliated with a fabulous curler which van der Sar saved. Scholes half-volleyed against the angle following an electrifying Giggs run, but

Ryan Giggs congratulates David Beckham on his stunning equaliser scored from a free-kick just after the half-hour

2 FULHAM

4, 48 SAHA

1. Edwin VAN DER SAR
2. Steve FINNAN
23. Sean DAVIS
4. Andy MELVILLE
24. Alain GOMA
14. Steed MALBRANQUE
7. Jon HARLEY
19. Bjarne GOLDBAEK
20. Louis SAHA
10. John COLLINS
15. Barry HAYLES

SUBSTITUTES

6. Kit SYMONS
12. Maik TAYLOR
25. Abdeslam QUADDOU (14) 88
26. Kevin BETSY (15) 84
40. Andrejs STOLCERS (19) 80

classy Fulham bounced back with both Saha and Hayles going close. When the equaliser came it was controversial: Beckham's free-kick was exquisite but the referee's ruling that Giggs had been fouled by Finnan looked extremely dubious. Before the interval Hayles was foiled by Barthez and Scholes by van der Sar, but there was no denying Saha after the break, when he raced on to Malbranque's perfect dispatch before netting with a 15-yard cross-shot.

Enter van Nistelrooy, first reacting quickly to bundle home from a Cole dink, then seizing on a rebound following a Beckham cross. From then on Fulham pressed forward bravely, forcing United – for whom Veron looked a little tentative – into an unexpected rearguard action. Three welcome points, then, but plenty of food for thought for Sir Alex Ferguson.

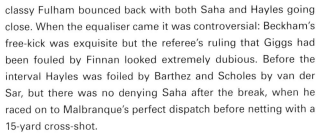
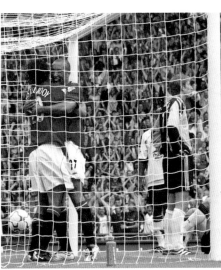
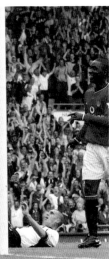

Ruud van Nistelrooy gets the plaudits after scoring his second goal in as many minutes

BLACKBURN ROVERS 2

1. Brad FRIEDEL
2. John CURTIS
16. Alan MAHON
4. Henning BERG
5. Stig Inge BJORNEBYE
6. Craig SHORT
7 . Garry FLITCROFT
18. Keith GILLESPIE
21. Corrado GRABBI
10. Matt JANSEN
11. Damien DUFF
SUBSTITUTES
12. Mark HUGHES
13. John FILAN
14. Nathan BLAKE (21) 74
15. Craig HIGNETT (18) 89
28. Martin TAYLOR (10) 79

BECKHAM (o.g.) 49
GILLESPIE 69

MATCH REPORT

The entertainment was compelling, the drama was ceaseless, as the action catapulted from end to end, and both sides, especially United, attacked with breathtakingly sumptuous flair. But after mounting a late rescue to salvage a draw from a contest which they had been dominating comprehensively, the Reds were left to rue another rickety defensive display. Stam and Gary Neville had been dropped in favour of Johnsen and Brown, but the opening sequences suggested that one soft centre had been exchanged for another as Gillespie drew a brilliant save from

Ryan Giggs is a study in concentration as he rounds off a beautiful move involving Roy Keane and Juan Sebastian Veron to give United the lead

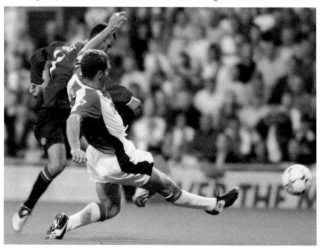

2   MANCHESTER UNITED

20 GIGGS
78 BECKHAM

1. Fabien BARTHEZ
27. Mikael SILVESTRE
3. Denis IRWIN
4. Juan Sebastian VERON
5. Ronny JOHNSEN
24. Wesley BROWN
7. David BECKHAM
18. Paul SCHOLES
16. Roy KEANE
10. Ruud VAN NISTELROOY
11. Ryan GIGGS
SUBSTITUTES
2. Gary NEVILLE (3) 69
9. Andy COLE (10) 74
13. Roy CARROLL
19. Dwight YORKE (18) 74
20. Ole Gunnar SOLSKJAER

Barthez, then Jansen headed against the bar. Blackburn continued to thrust brightly and Grabbi miscued horribly from close range after 19 minutes, but then United turned the tables with a move of utter beauty which began in midfield with Giggs, then continued through Keane and the majestic Veron, whose perfect through-ball set up the scurrying Welshman for an unstoppable 12-yard drive.

For the rest of the half, United played football fit for the gods, including two 30-yard efforts from Beckham and Scholes which were fingertipped against the woodwork by the fabulous Friedel. But Rovers refused to capitulate and levelled soon after the break when Mahon's cross skimmed Beckham's skull before eluding Barthez. Shortly afterwards, Berg crashed a header against the Reds' bar, then the French keeper narrowly escaped punishment from Grabbi after dallying dubiously on the ball. Now both sides attacked freely until Blackburn inched ahead when Gillespie lost Silvestre and buried an explosive left-footer on the turn.

The scales appeared to swing United's way when Short was dismissed for a second bookable offence and from the resultant free-kick Beckham chipped a controversial 35-yard equaliser before either Friedel or his wall were ready. But Rovers survived an 18-minute siege to share the spoils from one of the most scintillating games in Premiership history.

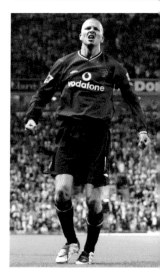

David Beckham's relief is palpable after chipping Brad Friedel with a 35-yard free-kick. Earlier he had diverted Mahon's cross into his own net

ASTON VILLA 1

1. Peter SCHMEICHEL	VASSELL 4
2. Mark DELANEY	
3. Alan WRIGHT	
4. Olof MELLBERG	
5. ALPAY Ozalan	
6. George BOATENG	
17. Lee HENDRIE	
8. Juan Pablo ANGEL	
22. Darius VASSELL	
10. Paul MERSON	
30. Hassan KACHLOUL	

SUBSTITUTES

12. Peter ENCKELMAN
14. David GINOLA
19. Bosko BALABAN (80) 78
20. Moustapha HADJI (10) 64
31. Jlloyd SAMUEL

MATCH REPORT

A frenzied late assault earned a deserved but seemingly unlikely point on a day of drama for the Red Devils. After conceding yet another early goal, it appeared that a pumped-up Peter Schmeichel was going to inflict defeat on his former employers as he blocked explosive late drives from Keane and van Nistelrooy. But deep into the third minute of added time, Giggs – on corner duty in place of Beckham, who had left the action with a groin strain – delivered a curling dispatch from the quadrant and Alpay, under severe pressure from Johnsen, headed past the fuming Dane. The equaliser offered welcome balm for the sizeable contingent of travelling fans still attempting to digest the day's bombshell news that world-class stopper Jaap Stam was to be sold to Lazio.

Certainly their concern about early-season defensive frailty had not been allayed by the manner in which Villa had sliced open the Reds' rearguard, Vassell bursting between Silvestre and Brown to stab home Kachloul's lovely left-wing cross from 12 yards. The goal offered a torrid welcome to the Premiership for new keeper Roy Carroll, deputising for the injured Barthez. Happily the Irishman was not fazed by that early reverse, going on to perform solidly and offer rich promise for the future.

Throughout a free-flowing game, the visitors enjoyed the majority of possession, with Veron passing beautifully, but their

Ronny Johnsen congratulates Ryan Giggs on his curling corner that was turned into his own net by Villa's Alpay

1 MANCHESTER UNITED

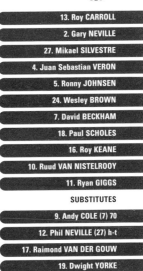

90 ALPAY (o.g.)

13. Roy CARROLL
2. Gary NEVILLE
27. Mikael SILVESTRE
4. Juan Sebastian VERON
5. Ronny JOHNSEN
24. Wesley BROWN
7. David BECKHAM
18. Paul SCHOLES
16. Roy KEANE
10. Ruud VAN NISTELROOY
11. Ryan GIGGS
SUBSTITUTES
9. Andy COLE (7) 70
12. Phil NEVILLE (27) h-t
17. Raimond VAN DER GOUW
19. Dwight YORKE
20. Ole Gunnar SOLSKJAER (18) 83

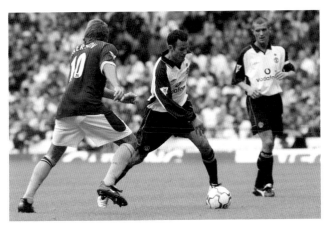

Roy Keane admires the delicate ball skills of Ryan Giggs as he dances his way past Paul Merson

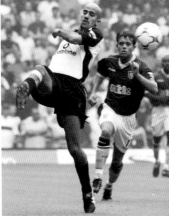

resultant goal attempts, including one bizarre free-kick which Beckham and Giggs appeared to take simultaneously, were either saved by Schmeichel or missed the target. United's best chance fell to van Nistelrooy after a thrilling run by Giggs but the Dutchman scooped over from six yards, while Villa might have doubled their lead before half-time when Carroll saved splendidly from Angel and only a fabulous tackle from Brown prevented Kachloul from converting the rebound. With Stam leaving, that was precisely the mettle young Wesley would be required to show in the months ahead.

Juan Sebastian Veron shows Villa's Lee Hendrie how it's done

AUGUST IN REVIEW

SUNDAY 19	v FULHAM	H	3-2
WEDNESDAY 22	v BLACKBURN ROVERS	A	2-2
SUNDAY 26	v ASTON VILLA	A	1-1

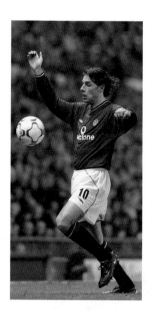

PLAYER IN THE FRAME

Ruud van Nistelrooy

Having cost some £19 million, and with his arrival at Old Trafford delayed for a year by a potentially career-threatening knee injury, the Dutch marksman found himself under immense instant pressure to succeed and he met the challenge magnificently. After scoring a classy goal in the Charity Shield, Ruud opened his Premiership account with a brace on his debut against Fulham, and despite being deployed frequently in the arduous role of lone striker, he never looked back.

FA BARCLAYCARD PREMIERSHIP

UP TO AND INCLUDING
SUNDAY 26 AUGUST 2001

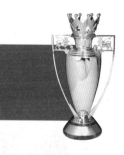

	P	W	D	L	F	A	Pts
Bolton Wanderers	3	3	0	0	8	1	9
Everton	3	2	1	0	5	2	7
Leeds United	3	2	1	0	4	1	7
Arsenal	3	2	0	1	9	2	6
MANCHESTER UNITED	3	1	2	0	6	5	5
Chelsea	2	1	1	0	3	1	4
Fulham	3	1	1	1	4	3	4
Blackburn Rovers	3	1	1	1	5	5	4
Derby County	3	1	1	1	3	4	4
Sunderland	3	1	1	1	2	3	4
Liverpool	2	1	0	1	3	3	3
Ipswich Town	3	1	0	2	3	3	3
Charlton Athletic	2	1	0	1	2	2	3
Newcastle United	2	0	2	0	2	2	2
Aston Villa	2	0	2	0	1	1	2
Tottenham Hotspur	3	0	2	1	2	3	2
West Ham United	2	0	1	1	1	2	1
Southampton	2	0	0	2	0	4	0
Middlesbrough	3	0	0	3	0	7	0
Leicester City	2	0	0	2	0	9	0

SEPTEMBER

SATURDAY 8	**v EVERTON**	**H**
SATURDAY 15	**v NEWCASTLE UNITED**	**A**
TUESDAY 18	**v LILLE OSC**	**H**
SATURDAY 22	**v IPSWICH TOWN**	**H**
TUESDAY 25	**v DEPORTIVO LA CORUÑA**	**A**
SATURDAY 29	**v TOTTENHAM HOTSPUR**	**A**

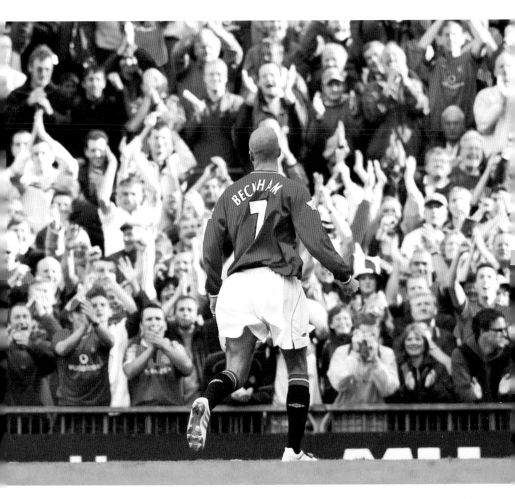

MANCHESTER UNITED 4

1. Fabien BARTHEZ
2. Gary NEVILLE
12. Phil NEVILLE
4. Juan Sebastian VERON
24. Wesley BROWN
6. Laurent BLANC
15. Luke CHADWICK
16. Roy KEANE
9. Andy COLE
19. Dwight YORKE
25. Quinton FORTUNE

SUBSTITUTES

7. David BECKHAM (15) 78
10. Ruud VAN NISTELROOY (19) 78
11. Ryan GIGGS
13. Roy CARROLL
27. Mikael SILVESTRE (2) 58

VERON 4
COLE 40
FORTUNE 46
BECKHAM 90

MATCH REPORT

A bewitchingly creative display by Juan Sebastian Veron was the centrepiece of the Red Devils' most fluent performance of the campaign to date. The Argentinian schemer orchestrated play with magisterial authority, destroying Everton with the accuracy and imagination of his passing and contributing a delicious opening goal for good measure. Meanwhile United's 35-year-old debutant, Laurent Blanc, slotted calmly into central defence, reading the game so effectively that the much vaunted physical threat of the Merseysiders' so-called 'Bruise Brothers', Ferguson and Campbell, was neutralised comprehensively.

Despite leaving Beckham, Giggs and van Nistelrooy on the bench and Scholes on the treatment table, the hosts began imperiously and Yorke almost gave them an early lead following a beautiful sweeping move instituted by Blanc and continued by Keane. Next the Tobagan set up Fortune for an instant 20-yard drive against the post, before the pressure paid off when Veron completed an exquisite one-two interchange with Keane, then chested the ball down and thrashed it past Gerrard from eight yards. United dominated the remainder of the half and went further ahead when Chadwick, who was on magnificent form, gulled two opponents and

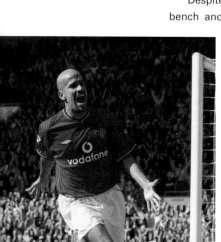

Juan Sebastian Veron is clearly delighted as he scores his first goal for United following a one-two with Roy Keane. Veron's performance was truly majestic

1 EVERTON

CAMPBELL 68

1. Paul GERRARD
2. Steve WATSON
3. Alessandro PISTONE
4. Alan STUBBS
5. David WEIR
6. David UNSWORTH
7. Niclas ALEXANDERSSON
17. Scot GEMMILL
9. Kevin CAMPBELL
10. Duncan FERGUSON
11. Mark PEMBRIDGE
SUBSTITUTES
13. Steve SIMONSEN
14. Idan TAL (4) 76
19. Joe-Max MOORE (7) 65
24. Abel XAVIER (5) 65
30. Nick CHADWICK

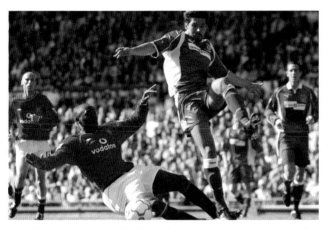

Andy Cole, who registered his first strike of the season just before half time, finds his way barred by Everton's Pistone

found Cole, who had only to clip into the far corner of an unguarded net from ten yards.

Moments after the restart Yorke nodded Gary Neville's long ball to the feet of the onrushing Fortune, who dinked deftly over Gerrard for the third goal. Everton might have folded, but they didn't and they regained a foothold when Campbell scrambled home from Gemmill's cross. Lifted by that, the visitors enjoyed their most influential spell and might have reduced the arrears still further when a Ferguson shot was deflected against a post.

Thus stung, United responded like champions, with van Nistelrooy and Veron going close before Beckham threaded a low 25-yarder past Gerrard to restore reality to the scoreline.

NEWCASTLE UNITED 4

1. Shay GIVEN
12. Andrew GRIFFIN
3. Robbie ELLIOT
4. Nolberto SOLANO
5. Andrew O'BRIEN
6. Clarence ACUNA
7. Robert LEE
34. Nikolas DABIZAS
9. Alan SHEARER
17. Craig BELLAMY
32. Laurent ROBERT

SUBSTITUTES

2. Warren BARTON (7) h-t
13. Steve HARPER
20. Lomana LUALUA
23. Shola AMEOBI
24. Sylvain DISTIN (17) 90

ROBERT 5
LEE 34
DABIZAS 52
SHEARER 82

MATCH REPORT

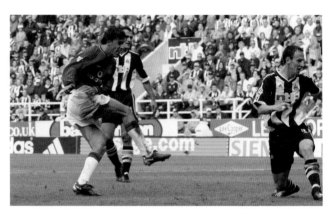

Perfect control, swivel and shot, sees Ruud van Nistelrooy equalise after Robert had given the Magpies an early lead

Manchester United suffered their first defeat of the season, the concession of four goals being compounded by the late dismissal of skipper Roy Keane. But even that triple dose of travail could not conceal the fact that, on a weekend when football needed to play a spirit-lifting part in the wake of the Manhattan atrocity, this was a fantastic match. Utterly irresistible going forward, serially vulnerable at the back, the Red Devils enchanted and frustrated alternately as the drama unfolded. It began when Blanc fouled Shearer, and Robert, the Magpies' overnight sensation, stepped up to curve home a dipping 25-yard free-kick of which Beckham would have been proud.

3 MANCHESTER UNITED

29 VAN NISTELROOY
62 GIGGS
64 VERON

1. Fabien BARTHEZ
2. Gary NEVILLE
12. Phil NEVILLE
4. Juan Sebastian VERON
24. Wesley BROWN
6. Laurent BLANC
7. David BECKHAM
16. Roy KEANE
9. Andy COLE
10. Ruud VAN NISTELROOY
11. Ryan GIGGS
SUBSTITUTES
5. Ronny JOHNSEN
8. Nicky BUTT
13. Roy CARROLL
18. Paul SCHOLES (9) 59
27. Mikael SILVESTRE

The visitors' response was an interlude of spellbindingly beautiful movement and passing in which the work of Veron, Beckham, Giggs and Keane was a wonder to behold, and it climaxed with a fabulous goal. Veron and Giggs weaved midfield magic, Gary Neville crossed and Cole nodded down to van Nistelrooy, whose control, swivel and shot were all faultless. However, Newcastle hit back and after being denied a penalty for a Phil Neville challenge on Bellamy, they regained the lead when a bouncing shot from Lee deceived Barthez. The Reds continued to make chances – van Nistelrooy alone might have scored four in the first half – but the hosts grabbed the next goal, too, Dabizas netting after a Robert drive had been blocked.

Now the Geordie hordes howled in triumph but soon they were silenced by two magnificent strikes in the space of two minutes, a rare right-footer from Giggs and a wonderful volley from the edge of the D by Veron. Thereafter the action see-sawed from end to end but the decisive strike was Shearer's, albeit with the aid of a couple of deflections. Even after that the excellent Scholes twice went agonisingly close to equalising, but it was not to be and the points remained at St James' Park.

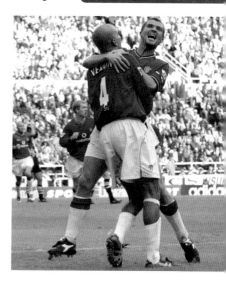

Skipper Roy Keane shows his delight after Juan Sebastian Veron's 64th-minute equaliser, but the Magpies had the last laugh as Shearer's late winner secured the points

MANCHESTER UNITED 1

1. Fabien BARTHEZ
2. Gary NEVILLE
3. Denis IRWIN
4. Juan Sebastian VERON
24. Wesley BROWN
6. Laurent BLANC
7. David BECKHAM
18. Paul SCHOLES
16. Roy KEANE
10. Ruud VAN NISTELROOY
11. Ryan GIGGS

SUBSTITUTES

5. Ronny JOHNSEN
8. Nicky BUTT
12. Phil NEVILLE
13. Roy CARROLL
19. Dwight YORKE
20. Ole Gunnar SOLSKJAER (11) 75
27. Mikael SILVESTRE (2) 12

BECKHAM 90

MATCH REPORT

The Red Devils kept their first clean sheet of the season but they needed a last-minute Beckham winner to ensure that Sir Alex Ferguson's latest tilt at Champions League glory got off to a winning start. Lille had been written off as makeweights in some quarters, but they had boasted a tighter defence than any club in Europe's five major domestic leagues last term, and their resilient, disciplined, occasionally inventive display at Old Trafford emphasised their stature as formidable opponents.

With Scholes operating once again as a deep-lying second striker, United mounted early pressure and might have nosed ahead following a slick link between Veron and van Nistelrooy, but the charging Dutchman failed to generate sufficient power of shot to trouble Wimbee. Then a luscious move climaxed with Giggs cutting in from the left before curling a right-footer narrowly wide of the far post. Van Nistelrooy and Scholes both went close as the hosts continued to buzz, but gradually the Frenchmen gained an attacking foothold and Barthez was forced to make a diving save from Cheyrou's free-kick, then pressurise Bakari into skying from the rebound.

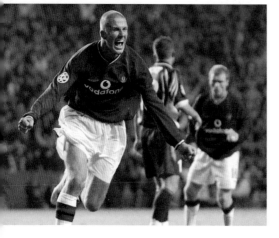

Fists clenched, David Beckham turns to celebrate his first Champions League goal of the season, and with good reason…

0 LILLE OSC

1. Gregory WIMBEE
18. Stephane PICHOT
3. Pascal CYGAN
4. Abdelilah FAHMI
20. Gregory TAFFOREAU
21. Johnny ECKER
19. Mile STERJOVSKI
27. Fernando Osvaldo D'AMICO
25. Sylvain N'DIAYE
10. Dagui Orphie BAKARI
28. Bruno CHEYROU
SUBSTITUTES
5. Rafael SCHMITZ (20) 86
9. Mikkel BECK
14. Adekanmi OLUFADE (19) 90
15. Djezon BOUTOILLE (28) 90
16. Eric ALLIBERT
22. Benoit CHEYROU
23. Mathieu DELPIERRE

Lille's resolution did not abate in the second half and, after Wimbee had fielded a Scholes scorcher, a deep Bakari cross almost deceived Barthez, who combined with Blanc to block the follow-up effort from Boutoille. United retaliated with a raking Beckham dispatch which was glanced on by van Nistelrooy to Solskjaer, whose firm volley was saved superbly by Wimbee.

As time ticked away Old Trafford oozed anxiety, but on 90 minutes Solskjaer nodded into the box, van Nistelrooy's shot was blocked, Scholes skipped over the loose ball and Beckham netted with a low shot. Still there was time for a fright as Brown left Ecker's cross, but Boutoille failed to find the empty net.

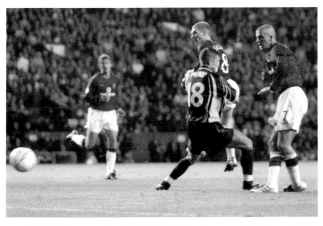

... with 90 minutes on the clock Paul Scholes jumps and Beckham strikes the winner to give United a great start to the new campaign

MANCHESTER UNITED 4

JOHNSEN 13
SOLSKJAER 20, 90
COLE 89

1. Fabien BARTHEZ
12. Phil NEVILLE
27. Mikael SILVESTRE
16. Roy KEANE
5. Ronny JOHNSEN
14. David MAY
15. Luke CHADWICK
8. Nicky BUTT
9. Andy COLE
20. Ole Gunnar SOLSKJAER
25. Quinton FORTUNE

SUBSTITUTES

2. Gary NEVILLE
4. Juan Sebastian VERON (16) 76
10. Ruud VAN NISTELROOY
13. Roy CARROLL
18. Paul SCHOLES (15) 64

MATCH REPORT

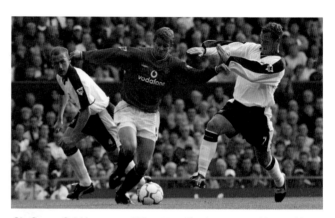

Ole Gunnar Solskjaer opened his account for the season with a goal in each half to ensure a crushing victory for United

Manchester United paraded an awesome show of force to the rest of the Premiership, not so much by the comfortable manner of their victory over last season's fifth-placed club, but by crushing Ipswich while resting no less than nine top players ahead of their Champions League clash with Deportivo La Coruña. True, May and Chadwick were the only uncapped Red Devils among Sir Alex Ferguson's starting combination,

Quinton Fortune is quickly on the scene to congratulate scorers Ole Gunnar Solskjaer and Andy Cole

0 IPSWICH TOWN

34. Matteo SERENI
2. Fabian WILNIS
15. Chris MAKIN
4. John McGREAL
5. Hermann HREIDARSSON
19. Titus BRAMBLE
7. Jim MAGILTON
8. Matthew HOLLAND
33. Finidi GEORGE
10. Alun ARMSTRONG
11. Marcus STEWART

SUBSTITUTES

3. Jamie CLAPHAM (15) 59
12. Richard NAYLOR
14. Jermaine WRIGHT (2) 75
21. Keith BRANAGAN
30. Martin REUSER (33) 59

and the visitors might have been a tad drained after completing a UEFA Cup tie only 41 hours earlier, but this was a mightily comprehensive manner in which to rotate any squad. The outcome seemed in no doubt after United struck twice in the first quarter. First the unmarked Johnsen headed in from a corner, then a lovely move instigated by Keane led to Sereni parrying Cole's low shot into the path of Solskjaer, who netted gleefully from close range. Ipswich's only retort before the interval was Stewart's stabbed effort which cleared the bar.

The pattern continued in the second period, with United exercising restrained superiority while their opponents laboured fruitlessly. The nearest George Burley's men came to registering was when Reuser broke free on the right and his raking delivery was met at point-blank range by the diving Stewart, only for Barthez to pull off a brilliant block.

The third goal was crafted by Scholes, whose through-pass to Cole freed the England man for a clinical finish, then another substitute midfielder, Veron, found Cole, who released the ball for Solskjaer to complete the rout from a narrow angle. The Norwegian sharpshooter admitted later that he had scored United's fourth with a mishit cross, setting the seal on a bad day for the East Anglians.

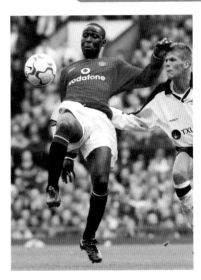

Andy Cole shows off his close control to Hreidarsson. The Ipswich defence were unable to cope with a rampant United

DEPORTIVO LA CORUÑA 2

1. Francisco MOLINA
2. MANUEL PABLO
3. Enrique ROMERO
4. Nourredine NAYBET
20. DONATO
6. MAURO SILVA
7. Roy MAKAAY
14. EMERSON
9. Diego TRISTAN
10. FRAN
16. SERGIO

SUBSTITUTES

11. Jose Emilio AMAVISCA
12. Lionel SCALONI (16) 61
13. NUNO Simoes
15. Joan CAPEDVILA
17. Walter PANDIANI (7) 61
19. Goran DJOROVIC
21. Juan Carlos VALERON (14) h-t

PANDIANI 86
NAYBET 90

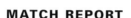

MATCH REPORT

It was so nearly the classic European performance as Manchester United soaked up relentless pressure from Deportivo and scored a fabulous goal on the break. But then, with only four minutes separating the seemingly composed Reds from their first away victory over Spanish opposition, they were shattered, cruelly and clinically, by two late strikes.

What made the reverse all the more demoralising was that United had fashioned enough chances in the second half to have put the result beyond doubt. They were missed, and the visitors found out how Bayern Munich must have felt some 28 months earlier in Barcelona. Anticipating a prolonged assault from Deportivo, Sir Alex Ferguson opted for a 4-1-4-1 formation, with Keane guarding the back four and van Nistelrooy operating as a lone striker. Duly the Spaniards spent most of the first period attacking fluently, with Fran and Tristan most prominent. However, Barthez and company were rarely

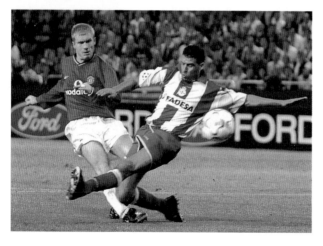

Paul Scholes thunders a rising drive into the Deportivo net to give United a well-deserved half-time lead

1 MANCHESTER UNITED

40 SCHOLES

1. Fabien BARTHEZ
2. Gary NEVILLE
3. Denis IRWIN
4. Juan Sebastian VERON
5. Ronny JOHNSEN
6. Laurent BLANC
7. David BECKHAM
18. Paul SCHOLES
16. Roy KEANE
10. Ruud VAN NISTELROOY
11. Ryan GIGGS

SUBSTITUTES

8. Nicky BUTT
9. Andy COLE (10) 90
12. Phil NEVILLE
13. Roy CARROLL
14. David MAY
20. Ole Gunnar SOLSKJAER (7) 90
27. Mikael SILVESTRE

stretched and Beckham found time for one ambitious soaring drive from his own half, reminiscent of his famous goal against Wimbledon. Then, shortly before the interval, the Reds made a nonsense of territorial disadvantage when Giggs broke out on the left and found Scholes, who exchanged passes with the excellent van Nistelrooy before thundering a rising drive past Molina from 14 yards.

After the break Deportivo swarmed forward again but the clearer openings fell to the visitors, Keane directing a 20-yard screamer straight at the keeper and Giggs shooting tamely from close range with only Molina to beat, albeit from a narrow angle. The sweet-passing Spaniards refused to panic, though, and United defended sluggishly as Valeron's scooped delivery was met by Pandiani, who netted from 12 yards, then Naybet was left unmarked to ram home a left-wing dispatch from a similar distance. It was an excruciating finale to an otherwise impeccably professional display by Sir Alex Ferguson's men.

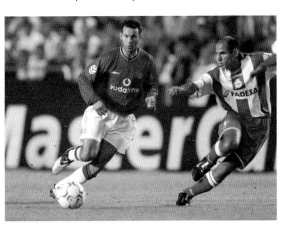

Despite second-half efforts from Ryan Giggs and Roy Keane, United were unable to add a second killer goal and were undone in four agonising minutes

TOTTENHAM HOTSPUR 3

1. Neil SULLIVAN	
26. Ledley KING	
3. Mauricio TARICCO	
4. Steffen FREUND	
36. Dean RICHARDS	
6. Chris PERRY	
7. Darren ANDERTON	
14. Gustavo POYET	
9. Les FERDINAND	
10. Teddy SHERINGHAM	
23. Christian ZIEGE	

SUBSTITUTES

11. Sergiy REBROV (7) 83
13. Kasey KELLER
28. Matthew ETHERINGTON
29. Simon DAVIES
31. Alton THELWELL

RICHARDS 15
FERDINAND 25
ZIEGE 45

MATCH REPORT

Even by the standards of Sir Alex Ferguson's famously resilient Reds, this was the stuff of footballing fantasy. Three goals down at the interval and staring a third successive defeat in the face, they roared back like some unstoppable force of nature to complete the most staggering revival in Premiership history.

After a slow start, Dean Richards, Tottenham's new £8 million defender, converted a Ziege corner with a stooping near-post header and Glenn Hoddle's side continued to counter-attack briskly, dominating the remainder of the half. Further goals came from Ferdinand, who slipped away from Blanc before beating Barthez with a venomous daisy-cutter, and Ziege, who was unmarked to net with a diving header from Poyet's cross.

Precisely what gentle words of encouragement were delivered by the manager at half-time remain firmly in the classified category, but suddenly there was renewed purpose in the visitors' play and it bore immediate fruit when Cole nodded in Gary Neville's inviting cross. Now, as the Reds hit their customary smooth-passing rhythm, the triumphalism which had engulfed White Hart Lane only minutes earlier was replaced by a palpable tremor of

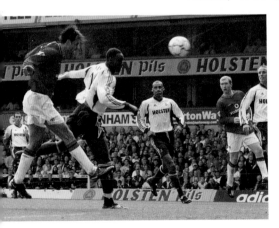

Goals from Andy Cole and Laurent Blanc, plus this thumping header from Ruud van Nistelrooy, restored parity at 3-3

5 MANCHESTER UNITED

46 COLE
58 BLANC
72 VAN NISTELROOY
76 VERON
87 BECKHAM

1. Fabien BARTHEZ
2. Gary NEVILLE
3. Denis IRWIN
4. Juan Sebastian VERON
5. Ronny JOHNSEN
6. Laurent BLANC
7. David BECKHAM
8. Nicky BUTT
9. Andy COLE
10. Ruud VAN NISTELROOY
18. Paul SCHOLES

SUBSTITUTES

12. Phil NEVILLE
13. Roy CARROLL
15. Luke CHADWICK
20. Ole Gunnar SOLSKJAER (8) 40
27. Mikael SILVESTRE (3) h-t

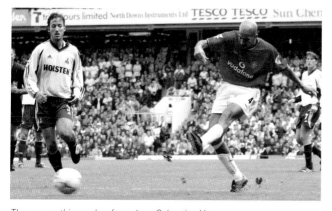

Then came this cracker from Juan Sebastian Veron ...

apprehension. Duly Spurs' roof fell in as a rampant United plundered four more goals. First Blanc rose high to register from a Beckham corner, then the head of van Nistelrooy met Silvestre's beautiful first-time dispatch to level the scores. Next came a sumptuous move culminating in the majestic Veron drilling home from 14 yards. All that remained was for Solskjaer to elude Taricco before finding Beckham unmarked on the edge of the box. The England captain's fierce half-volley was conclusive, a fitting climax to an unforgettable afternoon.

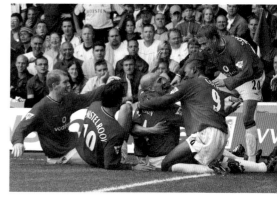

... and how they loved it!

SEPTEMBER IN REVIEW

SATURDAY 8	v EVERTON	H	4-1
SATURDAY 15	v NEWCASTLE UNITED	A	3-4
TUESDAY 18	v LILLE OSC	H	1-0
SATURDAY 22	v IPSWICH TOWN	H	4-0
TUESDAY 25	v DEPORTIVO LA CORUÑA	A	1-2
SATURDAY 29	v TOTTENHAM HOTSPUR	A	5-3

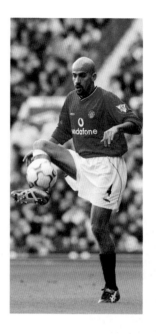

PLAYER IN THE FRAME

Juan Sebastian Veron

The Argentinian play-maker arrived with a reputation as one of the world's greatest footballers, and lost little time in justifying it. At this point, despite having had little time to integrate with his new team-mates, the Premiership's player of the month took the breath away with the vision and accuracy of his passing. In addition he scored wonderful goals against Everton and Newcastle, and there seemed no limit to what he might achieve as a Red Devil.

FA BARCLAYCARD PREMIERSHIP

UP TO AND INCLUDING
SATURDAY 29 SEPTEMBER 2001

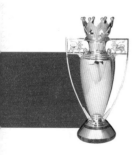

	P	W	D	L	F	A	Pts
Arsenal	7	4	2	1	16	5	14
MANCHESTER UNITED	7	4	2	1	22	13	14
Leeds United	6	4	2	0	9	1	14
Bolton Wanderers	8	3	3	2	10	6	12
Sunderland	8	3	3	2	8	7	12
Newcastle United	6	3	2	1	11	9	11
Everton	7	3	1	3	12	10	10
Aston Villa	5	2	3	0	7	3	9
Chelsea	5	2	3	0	9	6	9
Liverpool	5	3	0	2	8	7	9
Blackburn Rovers	7	2	3	2	8	8	9
Charlton Athletic	6	2	2	2	7	7	8
Tottenham Hotspur	8	2	2	4	11	13	8
Middlesbrough	8	2	1	5	8	17	7
Fulham	6	1	3	2	6	7	6
Southampton	6	2	0	4	5	10	6
Ipswich Town	6	1	2	3	5	9	5
West Ham United	6	1	2	3	4	9	5
Derby County	7	1	2	4	5	12	5
Leicester City	8	1	2	5	5	17	5

OCTOBER

WEDNESDAY 10	v OLYMPIAKOS PIRAEUS	A
SATURDAY 13	v SUNDERLAND	A
WEDNESDAY 18	v DEPORTIVO LA CORUÑA	H
SATURDAY 20	v BOLTON WANDERERS	H
TUESDAY 23	v OLYMPIAKOS PIRAEUS	H
SATURDAY 27	v LEEDS UNITED	H
WEDNESDAY 31	v LILLE OSC	A

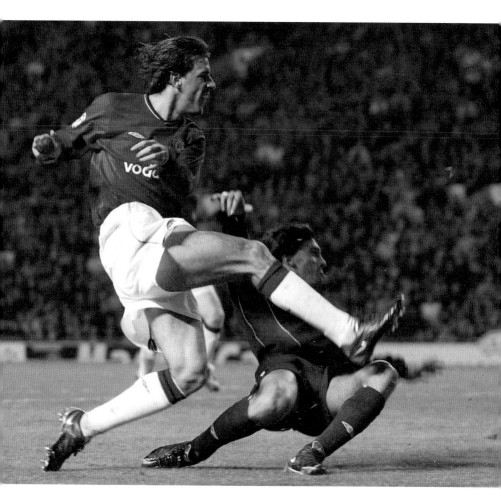

OLYMPIAKOS PIRAEUS   0

- 31. Dimitrios ELEFTHEROPOULOS
- 2. Christos PATSATZOGLOU
- 33. Stylianos VENETIDIS
- 4. Jorge BERMUDEZ
- 19. Athanasios KOSTOULAS
- 32. Georgios ANATOLAKIS
- 7. Stylianos GIANNAKOPOULOS
- 8. Christian KAREMBEU
- 20. Par Johan ZETTERBERG
- 10. GIOVANNI
- 11. Predrag DJORDJEVIC

SUBSTITUTES

- 5. Georgios AMANATIDIS
- 14. Dimitrios MAVROGENIDIS
- 15. Angelos GEORGIOU
- 17. Peter OFORIQUAYE (19) 70
- 21. Andreas NINIADIS (20) 66
- 24. Zizi ROBERTS
- 30. Alexios ALEXANDRIS (11) 80

MATCH REPORT

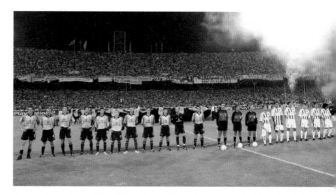

As usual, the fans at the Spiros Louis did their best to intimidate the visitors

Wearing gold for the first time in serious competition, the Red Devils gave their most lustrous performance on foreign soil since the glorious spring of 1999, condemning Olympiakos to their first ever home defeat in the Champions League. In truth the two-goal margin didn't reflect United's eventual superiority over the talented Greeks, who caused their visitors some anxiety at dead-ball situations in the first period, but were utterly outclassed in the second.

England's King David garnered yet more headlines by contributing the breakthrough goal

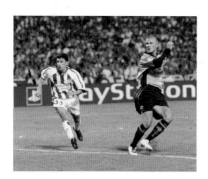

But two goals in the second half, the first from David Beckham...

2 MANCHESTER UNITED

66 BECKHAM
82 COLE

1. Fabien BARTHEZ
2. Gary NEVILLE
3. Denis IRWIN
4. Juan Sebastian VERON
5. Ronny JOHNSEN
6. Laurent BLANC
7. David BECKHAM
18. Paul SCHOLES
16. Roy KEANE
10. Ruud VAN NISTELROOY
11. Ryan GIGGS

SUBSTITUTES

9. Andy COLE (4) 80
12. Phil NEVILLE
13. Roy CARROLL
15. Luke CHADWICK
20. Ole Gunnar SOLSKJAER (10) 85
24. Wesley BROWN
27. Mikael SILVESTRE

but the most eye-catching performers were new boys Veron and van Nistelrooy. The Argentinian staged a breathtaking exhibition of matchlessly imaginative and uncannily accurate passing, while the unselfish Dutchman excelled in his thankless task of solitary spearhead.

United began by stroking the ball around in assured fashion, but appeared vulnerable whenever Djordjevic had a stationary ball at his feet. Karembeu went close with a near-post nod from a corner, Giannakopoulos headed over from a free-kick, then the Yugoslavian himself skimmed the bar from 25 yards. But the closest Olympiakos came to taking the lead was when Djordjevic swung in a 28th-minute free-kick which Giannakopoulos volleyed from point blank range, bringing a match-turning save from Barthez. Two minutes later Beckham and Giggs created the Reds' best chance of the half only for Veron to sidefoot wide from 15 yards, then the 'Little Witch' saw a fierce cross shot saved by Eleftheropoulos.

Come the second half United seized control, and after a Blanc header was cleared off the line by Karembeu, they took a deserved lead when Giggs' cutback from the byline was met with a precise Beckham half-volley from six yards. Thereafter the Reds dominated. Giggs and Blanc almost doubled the margin, then van Nistelrooy struck a post with a delicious curler before a Cole side-foot made the points safe after a sweet interchange with the Dutchman.

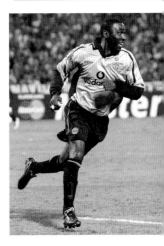

... and the second from Andy Cole sealed a memorable victory

SUNDERLAND 1

1. Thomas SORENSEN
18. Darren WILLIAMS
3. Michael GRAY
17. Jody CRADDOCK
5. Stanislav VARGA
21. Paul THIRLWELL
33. Julio ARCA
20. Stefan SCHWARZ
9. Niall QUINN
10. Kevin PHILLIPS
11. Kevin KILBANE

SUBSTITUTES

7. Lilian LASLANDES
14. Nicholas MEDINA
15. David BELLION (11) h-t
24. George McCARTNEY
30. Jurgen MACHO

PHILLIPS 83

MATCH REPORT

No Beckham, no Veron, no Keane, no van Nistelrooy, no Barthez... no matter. Still United were imperious as they stormed one of the most daunting of all Premiership citadels, making a formidable Sunderland side look distinctly ordinary in the process. With roving right-flanker Chadwick in scintillating form as the England captain's understudy, the Red Devils scaled the Black Cats with a performance of sustained precision and perception, and they might easily have doubled their victory tally. The tone for an unexpectedly one-sided encounter was set as early as the fifth minute when Solskjaer sent in Scholes, only for the excellent Sorensen to pull off the first of many fine saves.

Thereafter, with Butt and Scholes controlling central midfield, it seemed only a matter of time before United gained the ascendancy, even though Kilbane and Phillips spurned half-chances for the hosts. When the breakthrough duly materialised it came as the result of a flowing interchange involving Chadwick, Solskjaer and Cole, culminating in Chadwick's cross being headed past his own keeper by the straining Varga. Desperately in need of inspiration, the Wearsiders introduced Bellion after the interval, and the youngster made a telling early impact, gliding delightfully past

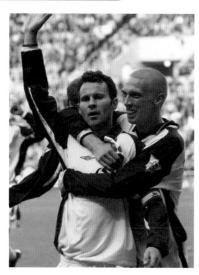

Luke Chadwick is first on the scene to congratulate Ryan Giggs on his 59th-minute goal

3 MANCHESTER UNITED

35 VARGA (o.g.)
59 GIGGS
66 COLE

13. Roy CARROLL	
2. Gary NEVILLE	
27. Mikael SILVESTRE	
18. Paul SCHOLES	
24. Wesley BROWN	
6. Laurent BLANC	
15. Luke CHADWICK	
8. Nicky BUTT	
9. Andy COLE	
20. Ole Gunnar SOLSKJAER	
11. Ryan GIGGS	
SUBSTITUTES	
10. Ruud VAN NISTELROOY	
12. Phil NEVILLE (6) 76	
17. Raimond VAN DER GOUW	
19. Dwight YORKE (11) 62	
28. Michael STEWART (18) 67	

Silvestre, Scholes and Brown before tumbling in the box, though he was not impeded. What followed was overwhelmingly one-sided. Solskjaer might have earned a penalty when he was floored by Bellion, but that was rendered irrelevant by two strikes midway through the half. First Giggs started a move inside his own half and sprinted forward to take Cole's perfect pass before stroking a crisp cross-shot past Sorensen, then Chadwick freed Cole and the England marksman, who had earlier struck a post, netted from 15 yards. Phillips salvaged respectability for Sunderland by sidestepping Carroll to score, but still the Reds dominated and a Yorke header hit the bar as the contest cruised towards its inevitable conclusion.

Sorensen, who made several excellent saves in the Sunderland goal, was unable to stop this sidefooter from Andy Cole that gave United a 3-0 lead

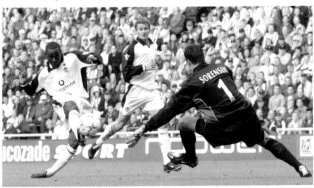

MANCHESTER UNITED 2

1. Fabien BARTHEZ

2. Gary NEVILLE

3. Denis IRWIN

4. Juan Sebastian VERON

5. Ronny JOHNSEN

6. Laurent BLANC

7. David BECKHAM

18. Paul SCHOLES

16. Roy KEANE

10. Ruud VAN NISTELROOY

11. Ryan GIGGS

SUBSTITUTES

8. Nicky BUTT

9. Andy COLE (18) 63

13. Roy CARROLL

15. Luke CHADWICK

20. Ole Gunnar SOLSKJAER (3) 85

24. Wesley BROWN (5) 8

27. Mikael SILVESTRE

VAN NISTELROOY 7, 40

MATCH REPORT

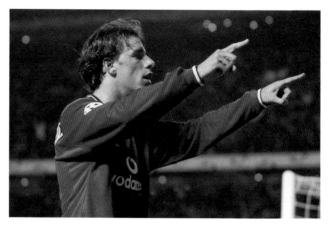

Two-goal van Nistelrooy celebrates, but this was not United's night

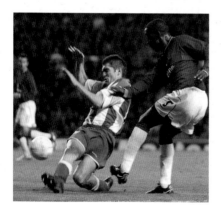

Even Andy Cole failed to score from several chances

This was a wonderful game, a richly exhilarating contest between two top-quality sides, but the bottom line is that Manchester United threw the points away. To be precise, the outrageously flamboyant but usually reliable Barthez gifted two goals to dazzling Deportivo, who needed no such charity to underline their pedigree as leaders of the Spanish League. That said, both teams crafted and missed a plethora of scoring opportunities and almost any result would have

3 DEPORTIVO LA CORUÑA

37 SERGIO
38, 60 TRISTAN

1. Francisco MOLINA
24. HECTOR
3. Enrico ROMERO
4. Nourredine NAYBET
20. DONATO
16. SERGIO
18. VICTOR Sanchez
23. Aldo Pedro DUSCHER
9. Diego TRISTAN
21. Juan Carlos VALERON
11. Jose Emilio AMAVISCA

SUBSTITUTES

5. CESAR
8. DJALMINHA
12. Lionel SCALONI
13. NUNO Simoes (1) h-t
14. EMERSON
15. Joan CAPDEVILA (3) 79
17. Walter PADIANI (9) 82

been possible. The pass-and-move football was unremittingly fluent from the early moment when Tristan eluded Johnsen but dinked tamely into the arms of Barthez. Soon United were in front thanks to a mazy and tenacious dribble by Giggs, who slipped the ball through for van Nistelrooy to net coolly from eight yards. Thereafter Deportivo surged forward and struck twice in quick succession. First the charging Barthez inexplicably failed to clear following a superb tackle by Brown and Sergio tapped in, then Tristan headed home from a Hector cross.

United's response was instant, van Nistelrooy burst into the box, shrugged off two defenders and deliciously scooped the ball past Molina from a narrow angle. Indeed, the Reds would have led by the interval had not Molina blocked a fierce Beckham drive. The second half was pulsating, with one phenomenal Barthez save from Valeron the early highlight. But then the Frenchman negated that by missing the ball after rushing from his line, allowing Tristan to find the empty net. United mounted a late blitz. Cole missed with a free header and van Nistelrooy shot over, but an equaliser refused to materialise and Deportivo leapfrogged the Reds to top the group.

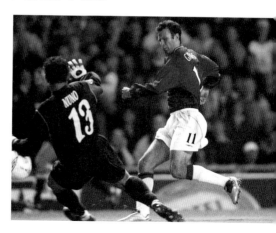

Ryan Giggs forces substitute keeper Nuno to save. The equaliser would not come

FA BARCLAYCARD PREMIERSHIP
Saturday 20 October, 2001

MANCHESTER UNITED   1

VERON 25

1. Fabien BARTHEZ
12. Phil NEVILLE
27. Mikael SILVESTRE
4. Juan Sebastian VERON
24. Wesley BROWN
14. David MAY
18. Paul SCHOLES
8. Nicky BUTT
9. Andy COLE
19. Dwight YORKE
20. Ole Gunnar SOLSKJAER

SUBSTITUTES

2. Gary NEVILLE (14) 78
11. Ryan GIGGS (18) 67
13. Roy CARROLL
15. Luke CHADWICK (19) 67
28. Michael STEWART

MATCH REPORT

For Manchester United, it was a demoralising end to a torrid week. Only three days after surrendering a lead and crashing to a home defeat against Deportivo, the below-par Reds suffered precisely the same fate against a gritty Bolton side which had emerged as the surprise package of the Premiership campaign.

Skippered by Scholes, who was making his 200th League appearance, and with a posse of stars rested with European commitments in mind, United began rather tentatively, although nothing could have been more emphatic than the manner in which they seized the lead.

Bergsson fouled Cole some 30 yards from goal and, with Beckham absent, up stepped Veron to curl home an exquisite free-kick of which the England captain would have been proud.

Now Old Trafford settled back in anticipation of a feast, but Bolton were in no mood to play the sacrificial lamb and they equalised spectacularly when N'Gotty floated a cross from the right, Ricketts headed down and Nolan left Barthez helpless with an explosive volley from the edge of the D. This spurred the hosts into action and for ten minutes the Reds hit their most compelling form of the afternoon, twice going close to regaining the

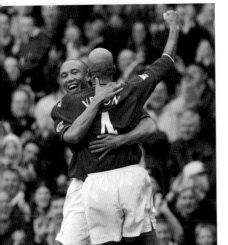

In David Beckham's absence, Juan Sebastian Veron was able to indulge himself with a 30-yard free kick of his own to give United a 25th-minute lead

2 BOLTON WANDERERS

35 NOLAN
84 RICKETTS

22. Jussi JAASKELAINEN
2. Bruno N'GOTTY
3. Mike WHITLOW
4. Gudni BERGSSON
25. Simon CHARLTON
6. Paul WARHURST
7. Bo HANSEN
8. Per FRANDSEN
17. Michael RICKETTS
15. Kevin NOLAN
11. Ricardo GARDNER

SUBSTITUTES

1. Steve BANKS
10. Dean HOLDSWORTH
21. Rod WALLACE
24. Anthony BARNESS (7) 83
28 Jermaine JOHNSON (6) 55

advantage. First Veron's 25-yarder was parried by Jaaskelainen to the feet of Solskjaer, who netted only to be judged offside; then the Bolton keeper pulled off two brilliant saves, from Scholes and the follow-up effort from Cole.

After the interval the Reds disappointed while the Trotters seemed to grow in stature, and there were chances at either end. Frandsen had a penalty claim rebuffed following a challenge by Veron, then the Argentinian shaved a post with a raking left-footer; Gardner went close for Bolton, Solskjaer for United – and so it went from end to end.

The decisive moment arrived when Brown misjudged a long clearance and the ball bounced to Ricketts, who advanced into the box before unleashing a rising drive which gave Barthez no chance. It was a fitting end to one of the performances of the season so far by anyone visiting Old Trafford.

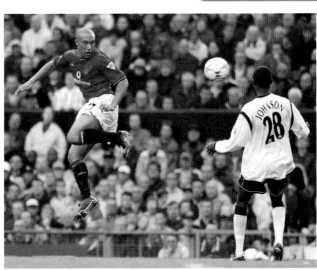

Mikael Silvestre jumps to clear from Bolton's Jermaine Johnson

MANCHESTER UNITED 3

| 1. Fabien BARTHEZ |
| 2. Gary NEVILLE |
| 3. Denis IRWIN |
| 4. Juan Sebastian VERON |
| 24. Wesley BROWN |
| 6. Laurent BLANC |
| 7. David BECKHAM |
| 8. Nicky BUTT |
| 18. Paul SCHOLES |
| 10. Ruud VAN NISTELROOY |
| 11. Ryan GIGGS |
| **SUBSTITUTES** |
| 12. Phil NEVILLE |
| 13. Roy CARROLL |
| 14. David MAY |
| 15. Luke CHADWICK |
| 19. Dwight YORKE |
| 20. Ole Gunnar SOLSKJAER (8) 72 |
| 27. Mikael SILVESTRE |

SOLSKJAER 80
GIGGS 88
VAN NISTELROOY 90

MATCH REPORT

Ole Gunnar Solskjaer, that rescue specialist extraordinaire, sparked a late goal rush which saw United progress to the second phase of the Champions League with a game to spare, but not before a pulsating contest had shredded the nerves of the Old Trafford faithful. Before the Norwegian sharpshooter struck, shortly after rising from the bench only 11 minutes before the final whistle, the Red Devils had surged forward with swashbuckling verve and fashioned a host of scoring opportunities. But as each one had been missed, the tension was racheted up another notch, especially as the home defence continued to look anything but secure and Olympiakos spurned several inviting openings.

The first meaningful blow in United's match-long battery was delivered by van Nistelrooy, whose powerful header from a Giggs cross was parried by Eleftheropoulos and Scholes almost forced home the rebound. Then Veron seized centre stage with characteristic flamboyance, trapping a flighted Beckham dispatch on his chest before dinking the ball over an opponent and drawing another smart save from the keeper with a crisp volley. Beckham shot into the side netting as the Reds continued to press, but Olympiakos responded by slicing through their hosts' soft centre with a long ball which freed Alexandris, only for the striker to delay so long that Blanc recovered to make a crucial challenge.

Down on his knees, but Ryan Giggs has just added United's second to put the game beyond the capable Olympiakos

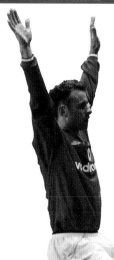

0 OLYMPIAKOS PIRAEUS

| 31. Dimitrios ELEFTHEROPOULOS |
| 2. Christos PATSATZOGLOU |
| 23. Christos KONTIS |
| 14. Dimitrios MAVROGENIDIS |
| 5. Georgios AMANATIDIS |
| 32. Georgios ANATOLAKIS |
| 7. Stylianos GIANNAKOPOULOS |
| 8. Christian KAREMBEU |
| 30. Alexios ALEXANDRIS |
| 17. Peter OFORIQUAYE |
| 11. Predrag DJORDJEVIC |

SUBSTITUTES

| 4. Jorge BERMUDEZ |
| 6. Ilias POURSANIDIS (14) h-t |
| 15. Angelos GEORGIOU |
| 19. Athanasios KOSTOULAS |
| 21. Andreas NINIADIS |
| 24. Zizi ROBERTS (7) 83 |
| 99. ALVEZ (30) 62 |

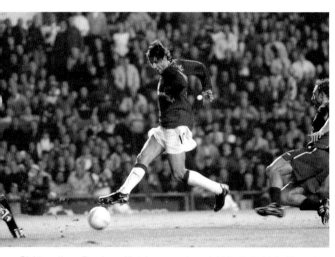

Right on time, Ruud van Nistelrooy cracks a right-foot shot into the net past Eleftheropoulos to round off a fine night for United

After the break United dominated and won a penalty for a foul on van Nistelrooy exacerbated by handball, but the Dutchman, who played magnificently throughout, saw his spot-kick saved athletically by Eleftheropoulos.

When Veron struck an upright with a 35-yard free-kick it seemed that the Reds were jinxed, but suddenly the Olympiakos dam broke. First van Nistelrooy played in Solskjaer, then sumptuous dispatches from Veron created the second and third goals for Giggs and van Nistelrooy. When Old Trafford duly erupted, the celebrations were tinged liberally with relief.

MANCHESTER UNITED 1

1. Fabien BARTHEZ

SOLSKJAER 89

2. Gary NEVILLE

27. Mikael SILVESTRE

4. Juan Sebastian VERON

24. Wesley BROWN

6. Laurent BLANC

7. David BECKHAM

8. Nicky BUTT

18. Paul SCHOLES

10. Ruud VAN NISTELROOY

11. Ryan GIGGS

SUBSTITUTES

12. Phil NEVILLE

13. Roy CARROLL

15. Luke CHADWICK

19. Dwight YORKE

20. Ole Gunnar SOLSKJAER (8) 75

MATCH REPORT

Seemingly doomed to defeat one minute, then so nearly snatching victory a few moments later, the Red Devils dragged their fans through a bewildering gamut of emotions when the League leaders paid a predictably tumultuous morning call on the champions. A game which had simmered entertainingly without truly igniting finally exploded in the closing stages. First Leeds edged in front when Viduka hooked home a Harte cross from what looked suspiciously like an offside position and at that point the visitors were on course for three points. But no task seems beyond Manchester United when Solskjaer prowls

Robbie Keane cracks a free-kick over the United wall and into the net only for the referee to rule that it had been taken prematurely

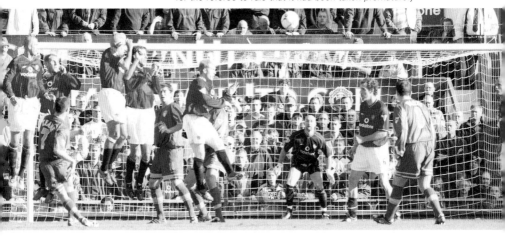

1   LEEDS UNITED

77 VIDUKA

1. Nigel MARTYN
18. Danny MILLS
3. Ian HARTE
4. Olivier DACOURT
29. Rio FERDINAND
21. Dominic MATTEO
7. Robbie KEANE
19. Eirik BAKKE
9. Mark VIDUKA
10. Harry KEWELL
11. Lee BOWYER

SUBSTITUTES

6. Jonathan WOODGATE
13. Paul ROBINSON
17. Alan SMITH (10) 90
20. Seth JOHNSON
23. David BATTY (7) 71

the pitch and yet again the Norwegian was the saviour, rising at the far post to head in a beautifully flighted centre from Giggs. Thus reprieved, the hosts eyed the bigger prize and they would have claimed it but for the reflexes of Martyn. First the England keeper clutched Matteo's netbound deflection from a Scholes dispatch, then he plunged full-length to repel van Nistelrooy's bullet header from a trademark Beckham delivery.

The Reds had dominated the first half-hour, creating a succession of scoring chances, but the visitors almost went ahead against the run of play when Viduka shot into the side-netting after being freed by Kewell. Gradually, though, Leeds gained the ascendancy and Kewell and Keane were both narrowly off-target with powerful drives as the first half ended. The Yorkshiremen continued to impress in the second period and on the hour Keane, who was lucky to be on the pitch after retaliating violently to a Beckham foul, netted with a glorious free-kick but the referee ruled that it had been taken prematurely. After that the action became more even, with near-misses by Keane at one end and Scholes at the other paving the way for that crackling climax.

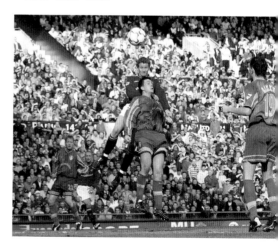

Ole Gunnar Solskjaer rises majestically to head in Ryan Giggs' cross for the equaliser

LILLE OSC 1

1. Gregory WIMBEE
18. Stephane PICHOT
3. Pascal CYGAN
4. Abdelilah FAHMI
15. Djezon BOUTOILLE
21. Johnny ECKER
19. Mile STERJOVSKI
27. Fernando Osvaldo D'AMICO
25. Sylvain N'DIAYE
12. Salaheddine BASSIR
28. Bruno CHEYROU

SUBSTITUTES

5. Rafael SCHMITZ
7. Edwin MURATI (12) 78
8. Patrick COLLOT
9. Mikkel BECK (15) 59
20. Gregory TAFFOREAU
24. Christophe LANDRIN (25) 86
26. Gregory MALICKI

CHEYROU 65

MATCH REPORT

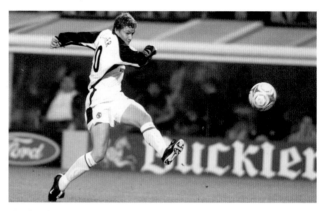

Ole Gunnar Solskjaer registers one of United's goals of the season, lashing home David Beckham's cross after six minutes

One of the great Manchester United goals, plundered by the red-hot Ole Gunnar Solskjaer, was not enough to secure leadership of their Champions League group, and with it a supposedly less daunting task in the next round.

In truth, ultra-competitive Lille deserved their draw in an eventful, high-octane clash with Sir Alex Ferguson's under-strength but still immensely talented and experienced combination, and despite the failure to attain his immediate objective, the United boss could reflect on plenty of positives from a night of high endeavour. In particular, there was a man-of-the-match performance from Silvestre, who was delighted to

1 MANCHESTER UNITED

6 SOLSKJAER

13. Roy CARROLL
12. Phil NEVILLE
3. Denis IRWIN
18. Paul SCHOLES
27. Mikael SILVESTRE
14. David MAY
7. David BECKHAM
8. Nicky BUTT
9. Andy COLE
20. Ole Gunnar SOLSKJAER
25. Quinton FORTUNE
SUBSTITUTES
15. Luke CHADWICK
17. Raimond VAN DER GOUW
19. Dwight YORKE (9) 76
22. Ronnie WALLWORK
28. Michael STEWART
30. John O'SHEA (14) 69
32. Bojan DJORDJIC

start in his preferred central defensive role; a hugely promising display from Carroll between the posts, and a composed European debut from rookie stopper O'Shea, who replaced May for the final quarter. First to take the eye was the Irish keeper, who came under intense scrutiny as Lille went for the Red Devils' throats from the off. He saved efficiently from Sterjovski after three minutes, then superbly from Bassir after four, and a siege seemed imminent.

But then the French were stunned by a moment of incandescent brilliance. A typically accurate Beckham dispatch located Solskjaer running behind the Lille backline, and the Norwegian lashed a rising drive across the helpless Wimbee and into the far top corner of the net from 15 yards. Now United assumed some measure of control and might have extended their advantage after 35 minutes when Wimbee leapt athletically to repel a Beckham free-kick. Lille remained feisty, though, and Ecker almost equalised when he shot wide from six yards on 42 minutes.

The French offensive resumed in the second half and the excellent Cheyrou brought a fabulous save from Carroll, then levelled the scores with a ferocious drive after eluding Butt and May. Thereafter Lille dominated territorially and merited the point which earned them a UEFA Cup berth.

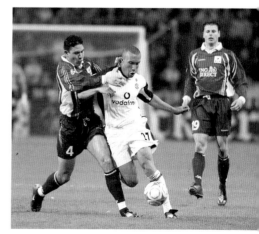

Man-of-the-Match Mikael Silvestre revelled in his favourite central defensive role

OCTOBER IN REVIEW

WEDNESDAY 10	v OLYMPIAKOS PIRAEUS	A	2-0
SATURDAY 13	v SUNDERLAND	A	3-1
WEDNESDAY 18	v DEPORTIVO LA CORUÑA	H	2-3
SATURDAY 20	v BOLTON WANDERERS	H	1-2
TUESDAY 23	v OLYMPIAKOS PIRAEUS	A	3-0
SATURDAY 27	v LEEDS UNITED	H	1-1
WEDNESDAY 31	v LILLE OSC	A	1-1

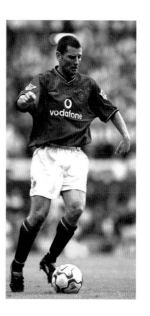

PLAYER IN THE FRAME

Denis Irwin

Though it was expected to be Denis's final season as a Red Devil, he remained a key contributor at the top level. His League appearances were sporadic, but he was ever-present in the first phase of the Champions League, his experience priceless in a rearguard which had yet to settle following the arrival of Laurent Blanc.

FA BARCLAYCARD PREMIERSHIP

UP TO AND INCLUDING
SATURDAY 27 OCTOBER 2001

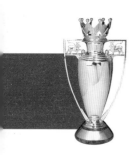

	P	W	D	L	F	A	Pts
Aston Villa	10	6	3	1	17	8	21
Leeds United	10	5	5	0	13	4	20
Arsenal	10	5	4	1	22	9	19
Liverpool	9	6	1	2	17	9	19
MANCHESTER UNITED	10	5	3	2	27	17	18
Newcastle United	10	5	2	3	18	14	17
Tottenham Hotspur	11	5	2	4	18	15	17
Bolton Wanderers	11	4	3	4	14	14	15
Chelsea	9	3	5	1	13	8	14
Everton	10	4	2	4	16	15	14
Blackburn Rovers	10	3	4	3	18	14	13
Sunderland	11	3	4	4	10	13	13
Fulham	10	2	5	3	10	12	11
Middlesbrough	11	3	2	6	11	19	11
West Ham United	9	3	2	4	9	17	11
Charlton Athletic	10	2	4	4	8	11	10
Ipswich Town	10	1	5	4	10	15	8
Southampton	10	2	1	7	9	19	7
Derby County	9	1	3	5	7	16	6
Leicester City	10	1	2	7	6	23	5

NOVEMBER

SUNDAY 4	v LIVERPOOL	A
MONDAY 5	v ARSENAL	A
SATURDAY 17	v LEICESTER CITY	H
TUESDAY 20	v BAYERN MUNICH	A
SUNDAY 25	v ARSENAL	A

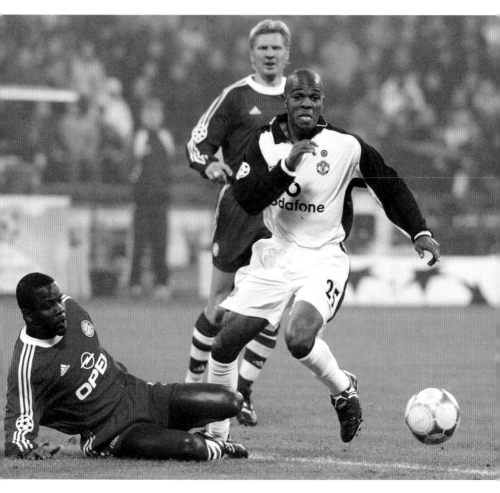

LIVERPOOL 3

OWEN 32, 51
RIISE 39

12. Jerzy DUDEK
2. Stephane HENCHOZ
18. John Arne RIISE
4. Sami HYYPIA
23. Jamie CARRAGHER
17. Steven GERRARD
7. Vladimir SMICER
8. Emile HESKEY
13. Danny MURPHY
10. Michael OWEN
16. Dietmar HAMANN

SUBSTITUTES

9. Robbie FOWLER (10) 69
11. Jamie REDKNAPP
15. Patrik BERGER (7) 69
22. Chris KIRKLAND
29. Stephen WRIGHT

MATCH REPORT

What was expected to be Sir Alex Ferguson's final League visit to Anfield ended in emphatic defeat. Worse, by the manager's own admission, was the stark truth that the Red Devils had surrendered tamely to their fiercest rivals. Ironically, United looked the more fluent side in the opening exchanges and after ten minutes van Nistelrooy was unlucky not to score. But gradually it became apparent that Liverpool were sharper, more purposeful and convincing, and inexorably they gained the upper hand. The first significant warning of the grief to follow came after quarter of an hour, when Smicer broke free on the left and his cross was met by Owen's 12-yard snap-volley, which was saved capably by Barthez.

However, the Frenchman had no chance when Brown's miskick under pressure from Heskey allowed another Smicer dispatch to reach Owen, who curled home an exquisite shot from the edge of the box. Then, with the visitors still reeling, Hamann touched a free-kick to Riise, whose 30-yard piledriver arrowed into the net via the crossbar. Now United needed an early second-half breakthrough, and it arrived when Riise misjudged an Irwin cross and Beckham pounced to score. However,

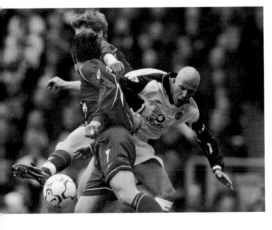

David Beckham is sandwiched between Liverpool's Riise and Smicer

1 MANCHESTER UNITED

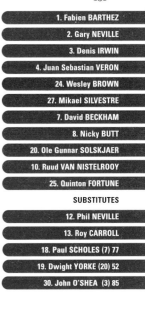

50 BECKHAM

1. Fabien BARTHEZ
2. Gary NEVILLE
3. Denis IRWIN
4. Juan Sebastian VERON
24. Wesley BROWN
27. Mikael SILVESTRE
7. David BECKHAM
8. Nicky BUTT
20. Ole Gunnar SOLSKJAER
10. Ruud VAN NISTELROOY
25. Quinton FORTUNE
SUBSTITUTES
12. Phil NEVILLE
13. Roy CARROLL
18. Paul SCHOLES (7) 77
19. Dwight YORKE (20) 52
30. John O'SHEA (3) 85

that hard-won impetus was squandered within 90 seconds when Barthez failed to claim a long-throw from Riise, Heskey headed on and Owen was left to nod into an empty net.

Thereafter the Red Devils dominated possession, but it was meaningless as only once did they create a decent opening, when a Beckham shot was saved smartly by the mostly under-employed Dudek after 67 minutes. Even the anticipated late assault failed to materialise, leaving the Liverpool fans to gloat 'Are you City in disguise?' as the champions trooped off disconsolately, a well-beaten team.

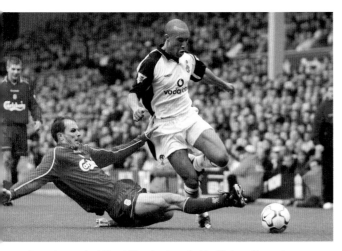

A surging run by Mikael Silvestre is ended by Dietmar Hamann

ARSENAL 4

24. Richard WRIGHT
22. Oleg LUZHNY
16. Giovanni VAN BRONCKHORST
27. Stathis TAVLARIDIS
26. Igors STEPANOVS
18. Gilles GRIMANDI
21. Jermaine PENNANT
15. Ray PARLOUR
25. Nwankwu KANU
17. EDU
11. Sylvain WILTORD

SUBSTITUTES

12. LAUREN
13. Stuart TAYLOR
36. John HALLS (16) h-t
37. Carlin ITONGA (18) 85
40. Rohan RICKETTS (21) 74

WILTORD 15, 30 (pen.), 45
KANU 67 (pen.)

MATCH REPORT

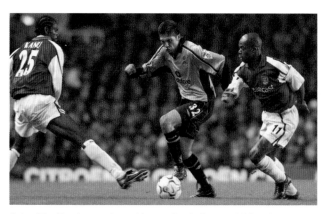

Bojan Djordjic takes on Arsenal internationals Kanu and Wiltord

It was men against boys as a team consisting mainly of Manchester United rookies was overwhelmed comfortably by Arsenal, who fielded eight full internationals. They included World Cup winner Sylvain Wiltord, who bagged a first-half hat-trick which ended the game as a meaningful contest. That said, there were plenty of pluses for the callow Red Devils, with Roche, Davis and Nardiello making their senior debuts, while O'Shea, Stewart, Djordjic and Webber are not exactly gnarled veterans and they benefited enormously from the experience. United battled spiritedly, and played some clever football at times, but were vulnerable to swift attacks through the centre, such as the move which led to the opening goal. Grimandi

0 MANCHESTER UNITED

13. Roy CARROLL	
34. Lee ROCHE	
12. Phil NEVILLE	
28. Michael STEWART	
30. John O'SHEA	
22. Ronnie WALLWORK	
15. Luke CHADWICK	
36.Jimmy DAVIS	
37. Danny WEBBER	
19. Dwight YORKE	
32. Bojan DJORDJIC	

SUBSTITUTES

17. Raimond VAN DER GOUW (13) h-t	
23. Michael CLEGG (22) 82	
39. Paul TIERNEY	
40. Daniel NARDIELLO (32) 72	
41. Alan TATE	

emerged from a midfield skirmish with the ball before slipping it to Kanu, who freed Wiltord to beat Carroll with clinical precision.

The visitors retaliated enterprisingly though, and might have equalised when Davis broke free on the right and set up the unmarked Djordjic for a 12-yard shot which flashed narrowly wide, then Wright was forced to save at the feet of the charging Webber. But soon the Gunners took charge, doubling their lead with a Wiltord penalty after Carroll had tripped Kanu, then trebling it when splendid work by Pennant and Parlour enabled Wiltord to control the ball on his forehead before flicking adroitly past Carroll to complete his hat-trick. Soon after the interval, substitute keeper van der Gouw saved superbly from Wiltord following a beautiful set-up by Edu, but it wasn't one-way traffic and Djordjic was woefully unlucky when his deflected free-kick was touched on to the crossbar by Wright.

Arsenal struck again when Wallwork tangled with Wiltord in the box and the referee awarded his second penalty of the night, Kanu converting the spot-kick with characteristic composure. All that remained was for Arsenal debutant Halls to be red-carded for a second bookable offence, a tackle from behind on Djordjic.

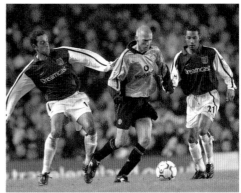

Luke Chadwick was unable to use his experience to spur the other United youngsters

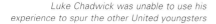

MANCHESTER UNITED 2

1. Fabien BARTHEZ
2. Gary NEVILLE
3. Denis IRWIN
16. Roy KEANE
24. Wesley BROWN
6. Laurent BLANC
7. David BECKHAM
18. Paul SCHOLES
19. Dwight YORKE
10. Ruud VAN NISTELROOY
11. Ryan GIGGS

SUBSTITUTES

8. Nicky BUTT
13. Roy CARROLL
20. Ole Gunnar SOLSKJAER
25. Quinton FORTUNE (11) 64
27. Mikael SILVESTRE (3) h-t

VAN NISTELROOY 21
YORKE 50

MATCH REPORT

Seldom in the past decade has a routine victory over Premiership strugglers been more welcome than the Red Devils' ultimately convincing triumph over Leicester. It was hardly a vintage performance, with one or two scares along the way, but it was enough to suggest that the recent torrent of obituaries to Sir Alex Ferguson's Old Trafford empire were a tad premature.

However, the United boss must have cringed at early evidence of uncertainty in his much-criticised rearguard. First Blanc's routine backpass was misdirected by Barthez to Akinbiyi, who could only fumble the ball back to the errant keeper; then the City spearhead eluded two markers only to head wide from a Benjamin cross. In between those escapes, though, there were

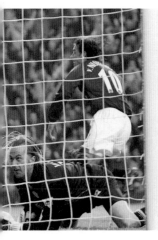

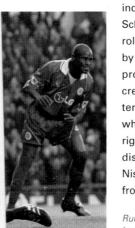

indications of a Reds resurgence and Scholes, thriving in his preferred midfield role, saw a trademark scorcher blocked by Sinclair. Though the visitors toiled prodigiously, the hosts' superior creativity enabled them to establish territorial dominance, which paid off when Keane found Beckham on the right and the England captain's arcing dispatch was converted by van Nistelrooy's powerful downward header from six yards.

Ruud van Nistelrooy turns away having beaten keeper Walker with a powerful header

0 LEICESTER CITY

16. Ian WALKER

26. Lee MARSHALL

3. Frank SINCLAIR

14. Callum DAVIDSON

18. Matthew ELLIOT

6. Muzzy IZZET

24. Andrew IMPEY

23. Jordan STEWART

20. Trevor BENJAMIN

22. Ade AKINBIYI

11. Dennis WISE

SUBSTITUTES

5. Alan ROGERS (14) h-t

7. Matthew JONES

10. Jamie SCOWCROFT (20) 57

12. Simon ROYCE

28. Matthew HEATH

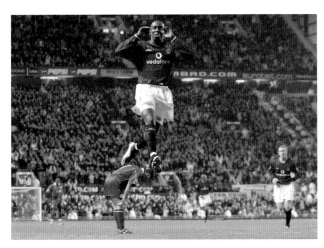

First of the season: Dwight Yorke leaps high to celebrate his goal

Moments later Blanc conceded a penalty, bundling over Benjamin, and setting the scene for the latest unorthodox Barthez interlude. As Izzet shaped for the spot-kick, the Frenchman leant idly against a post; the whistle sounded, Izzet rolled the ball into the empty net and a retake was ordered. This time Barthez dived to divert a low shot against an upright and away to safety.

Thereafter United dominated and just before the interval van Nistelrooy hit the post from a Beckham cross only for Keane to nod wide from the rebound. Soon, though, Yorke doubled the lead with a flashing header from Neville's cross, then Giggs struck the bar with an exquisite curler.

Normal service? Not quite, but the signs were encouraging.

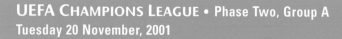

BAYERN MUNICH   1

PAULO SERGIO 87

1. Oliver KAHN
2. Willy SAGNOL
3. Bixente LIZARAZU
4. Samuel Osei KUFFOUR
12. Robert KOVAC
20. Hasan SALIHAMIDZIC
14. Claudio PIZARRO
23. Owen HARGREAVES
9. Giovane ELBER
13. PAULO SERGIO
11. Stefan EFFENBERG

SUBSTITUTES

10. Ciriaco SFORZA (11) 67
17. Thorsteen FINK
18. Michael TARNAT
19. Carsten JANCKER (9) 67
21. Alexander ZICKLER (2) 73
25. Thomas LINKE

MATCH REPORT

Manchester United fans didn't know whether to celebrate or reach for the sackcloth and ashes when the final whistle ended a tautly compelling encounter with the European champions. On the positive side, Sir Alex Ferguson's men had confounded predictions of an imminent thrashing and claimed a precious point, but the achievement was marred by a late Bayern goal which deprived them of a famous victory.

In the first half United defended with iron discipline, limiting Bayern to a succession of half chances. Irwin nodded a near-post Salihamidzic header off the line, Hargreaves' follow-up drive was deflected wide and Salihamidzic just failed to turn

David Beckham worked tirelessly in a tight midfield

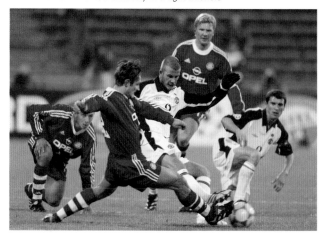

1 MANCHESTER UNITED

74 VAN NISTELROOY

home an Effenberg free-kick. Fortune, deputising for hamstring victim Giggs, came closest at the other end, his header from a Beckham dispatch bouncing past an upright. After the break, though the Germans continued to enjoy territorial superiority, the Reds were more adventurous and they reaped a rich reward when Scholes freed Silvestre down the left and the Frenchman curled an exquisite cross around two defenders for van Nistelrooy to volley beyond Kahn from five yards.

Now Bayern were clearly rattled and Keane came agonisingly close to sealing a win, only for Kahn to fingertip the Irishman's 20-yard screamer against the crossbar. But the Reds were undone three minutes from time when an apparently harmless through-pass took a deflection, thus wrong-footing Silvestre. The ball ran to Paulo Sergio, who netted with ease. The situation could have worsened when Sforza shot fiercely from 16 yards, but Barthez rescued the Reds with a fine save. Nerve-wracking stuff, but students of United-Bayern games will not have been surprised by a touch of late drama.

1. Fabien BARTHEZ
2. Gary NEVILLE
3. Denis IRWIN
4. Juan Sebastian VERON
24. Wesley BROWN
6. Laurent BLANC
7. David BECKHAM
18. Paul SCHOLES
16. Roy KEANE
10. Ruud VAN NISTELROOY
25. Quinton FORTUNE
SUBSTITUTES
8. Nicky BUTT
12. Phil NEVILLE
13. Roy CARROLL
15. Luke CHADWICK
19. Dwight YORKE (10) 85
20. Ole Gunnar SOLSKJAER
27. Mikael SILVESTRE (3) h-t

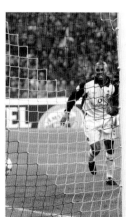
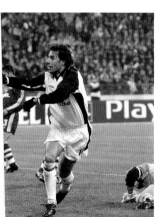

Ruud van Nistelrooy puts United ahead from Silvestre's superb cross

ARSENAL 3

13. Stuart TAYLOR
12. LAUREN
3. Ashley COLE
4. Patrick VIEIRA
23. Sol CAMPBELL
20. Matthew UPSON
7. Robert PIRES
8. Fredrik LJUNGBERG
25. Nwankwu KANU
15. Ray PARLOUR
14. Thierry HENRY

SUBSTITUTES

10. Dennis BERGKAMP (25) 64
11. Sylvain WILTORD
16. Giovanni VAN BRONCKHORST
18. Gilles GRIMANDI (7) 83
43. Graham STACK

LJUNGBERG 49
HENRY 80, 85

MATCH REPORT

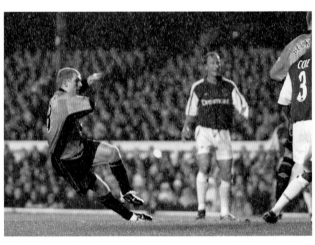

Paul Scholes registers his first goal of the season to put United ahead...

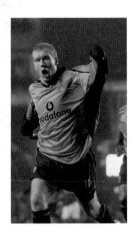

Ten minutes from time, Fabien Barthez was odds-on to be man of the match after his series of brilliant saves had kept the Red Devils in contention in a frenetic encounter largely dominated by Arsenal. But then the sky fell in on the flamboyant Frenchman, who proceeded to gift the points to the Gunners with two grotesque blunders, both of which resulted in goals by Henry. The late melodrama made for a grisly climax to an afternoon of starkly contrasting emotions for United's legion of travelling fans. It had begun with apprehension as the gold-

...and looks suitably pleased with himself

1 MANCHESTER UNITED

14 SCHOLES

1. Fabien BARTHEZ
2. Gary NEVILLE
27. Mikael SILVESTRE
4. Juan Sebastian VERON
24. Wesley BROWN
6. Laurent BLANC
7. David BECKHAM
18. Paul SCHOLES
16. Roy KEANE
10. Ruud VAN NISTELROOY
25. Quinton FORTUNE

SUBSTITUTES

8. Nicky BUTT
12. Phil NEVILLE (27) 57
13. Roy CARROLL
19. Dwight YORKE (4) 58
20. Ole Gunnar SOLSKJAER (10) 78

shirted Reds were forced to weather early pressure, with Barthez fisting a free-kick by Henry over his bar. But soon the mood switched to exultation as a slick move involving Fortune, Scholes and van Nistelrooy resulted in Silvestre wrong-footing Lauren, then crossing from the left for Scholes to sweep home from seven yards, his first strike of the Premiership campaign.

Gradually, though, the hosts assumed territorial supremacy, with Barthez saving smartly from Pires, Parlour and Henry before half-time. Shortly after the interval Arsenal claimed a deserved equaliser when Gary Neville's slack pass was intercepted by Pires, who set up Ljungberg to score with an exquisitely judged 18-yard chip. Thereafter the Red Devils were engulfed by a non-stop wave of attacks, while offering precious little in return. As the pressure mounted, Henry had two penalty claims turned down.

The Gunners continued to fashion chance after chance, only to be denied each time by Barthez. He saved athletically from Kanu, fielded a header from Henry, blocked his countryman in a one-on-one, then held a snap-volley from Pires. How cruelly ironic, then, that Barthez should be the instrument of United's downfall. First he scuffed a routine clearance, then fumbled a long ball from Vieira, both times allowing Henry to net at his leisure.

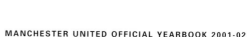

So near yet so far: Fabien Barthez can't believe that his great performance could end so badly

NOVEMBER IN REVIEW

SUNDAY 4	v LIVERPOOL	A	1-3
MONDAY 5	v ARSENAL	A	0-4
SATURDAY 17	v LEICESTER CITY	H	2-0
TUESDAY 20	v BAYERN MUNICH	A	1-1
SUNDAY 25	v ARSENAL	A	1-3

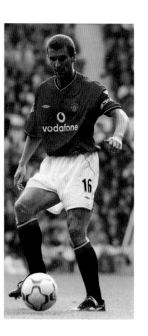

PLAYER IN THE FRAME

Roy Keane

At a point in the campaign when the going became unexpectedly tough for the Red Devils, skipper Roy Keane stood up to be counted. Clearly enraged at the turn events were taking, the Irishman was more influential than ever, often appearing to lift his team-mates by sheer force of will, tackling, passing, running and exhorting the rest to greater effort with every shred of his being. But for Roy's steel and passion, the Reds' season might have sunk without trace.

FA BARCLAYCARD PREMIERSHIP

UP TO AND INCLUDING
WEDNESDAY 29 NOVEMBER 2001

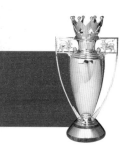

	P	W	D	L	F	A	Pts
Liverpool	12	8	2	2	22	11	28
Leeds United	13	6	6	1	16	8	24
Arsenal	13	6	5	2	28	15	23
Newcastle United	13	7	2	4	23	17	23
Aston Villa	13	6	5	2	18	12	23
MANCHESTER UNITED	13	6	3	4	31	23	21
Tottenham Hotspur	14	6	3	5	21	18	21
Chelsea	13	4	8	1	16	11	20
Bolton Wanderers	14	5	5	4	18	17	20
Blackburn Rovers	14	4	7	3	21	16	19
Fulham	13	4	6	3	15	13	18
Everton	13	4	5	4	18	17	17
Sunderland	14	4	4	6	12	15	16
Middlesbrough	14	4	4	6	16	20	16
West Ham United	13	4	3	6	16	26	15
Charlton Athletic	13	3	5	5	16	18	14
Southampton	13	3	1	9	11	22	10
Derby County	13	2	4	7	10	23	10
Leicester City	14	2	4	8	7	25	10
Ipswich Town	14	1	6	7	14	22	9

DECEMBER

SATURDAY 1	v CHELSEA	H
WEDNESDAY 5	v BOAVISTA	H
SATURDAY 8	v WEST HAM UNITED	H
WEDNESDAY 12	v DERBY COUNTY	H
SATURDAY 15	v MIDDLESBROUGH	A
SATURDAY 22	v SOUTHAMPTON	H
WEDNESDAY 26	v EVERTON	A
SUNDAY 30	v FULHAM	A

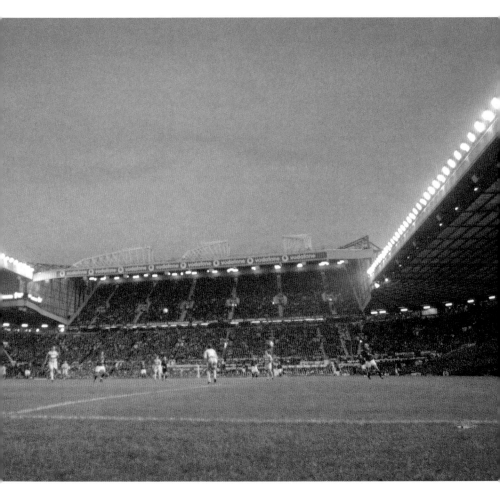

MANCHESTER UNITED   0

1. Fabien BARTHEZ
24. Wesley BROWN
12. Phil NEVILLE
4. Juan Sebastian VERON
16. Roy KEANE
6. Laurent BLANC
7. David BECKHAM
18. Paul SCHOLES
9. Andy COLE
10. Ruud VAN NISTELROOY
25. Quinton FORTUNE

SUBSTITUTES

2. Gary NEVILLE (25) 67
13. Roy CARROLL
15. Luke CHADWICK (9) 90
20. Ole Gunnar SOLSKJAER (7) 76
27. Mikael SILVESTRE

MATCH REPORT

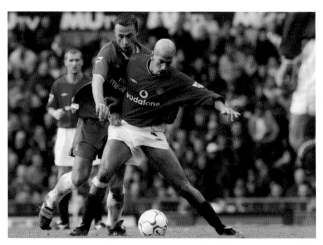

Juan Sebastian Veron pushes off Chelsea's Slavisa Jokanovic

Let's be honest. By their own lofty standards, Manchester United were woeful against a polished Chelsea team who outplayed them for all but the first five minutes of each half. The comprehensive defeat, which would have been even more emphatic but for the Londoners' erratic finishing, was the Red Devils' fifth reverse of the Premiership campaign and left their dreams of a fourth successive title looking sadly forlorn.

As a reaction to previous setbacks, the champions began with a radically reshuffled rearguard, with Keane partnering Blanc in the centre and Brown shifting to right-back, but the ploy was

3 CHELSEA

6 MELCHIOT
64 HASSELBAINK
86 GUDJOHNSEN

23. Carlo CUDICINI
15. Mario MELCHIOT
3. Celestine BABAYARO
13. William GALLAS
26. John TERRY
14. Graham LE SAUX
24. Sam DALLA BONA
8. Frank LAMPARD
9. Jimmy Floyd HASSELBAINK
10. Slavisa JOKANOVIC
22. Eidur GUDJOHNSEN
SUBSTITUTES
1. Ed DE GOEY
11. Boudewijn ZENDEN
12. Mario STANIC (14) 84
25. Gianfranco ZOLA (22) 88
32. Mikael FORSSELL (9) 82

abandoned during a second half in which Chelsea were rampant. Maybe, just maybe, the outcome might have been different if Sir Alex Ferguson's men had made the most of a bright start when van Nistelrooy struck a venomous volley from ten yards, only for the ball to bounce to safety off the knee of the diving Cudicini. Thereafter, the news was all bad. The visitors took the lead when Melchiot eluded Brown to net with a thumping header from Hasselbaink's left-wing corner, and then they seized command, taking advantage of their hosts' uncharacteristic lack of conviction. Gudjohnsen set up opportunities for Hasselbaink and Dalla Bona but both were spurned, then Le Saux twanged the crossbar with a 25-yard half-volley.

Veron went close with a free-kick just before the interval but, after surviving the Reds' brisk opening to the second period, the Blues underlined their supremacy when Hasselbaink swapped passes with Gudjohnsen and drilled a fierce shot past Barthez.

Scholes hit back with a 45-yard chip which Gallas cleared off his line, but when Gudjohnsen sprang United's lethargic offside trap to make it three, there could be no arguing with the justice of the final scoreline.

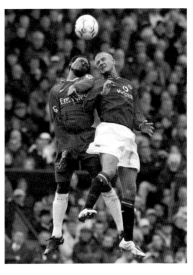

David Beckham lifts off in an effort to challenge Chelsea's Nigerian international Celestine Babayaro

MANCHESTER UNITED 3

1. Fabien BARTHEZ

2. Gary NEVILLE

27. Mikael SILVESTRE

4. Juan Sebastian VERON

12. Phil NEVILLE

6. Laurent BLANC

16. Roy KEANE

8. Nicky BUTT

19. Dwight YORKE

10. Ruud VAN NISTELROOY

18. Paul SCHOLES

SUBSTITUTES

7. David BECKHAM

13. Roy CARROLL

15. Luke CHADWICK

20. Ole Gunnar SOLSKJAER (10) 88

22. Ronnie WALLWORK

25. Quinton FORTUNE (18) 86

30. John O'SHEA (2) 77

VAN NISTELROOY 31, 62
BLANC 55

MATCH REPORT

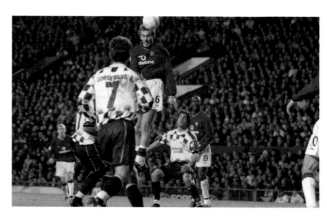

Unmarked, Laurent Blanc rises to head home Juan Sebastian Veron's corner in the 55th minute

Four days after their abject capitulation to Chelsea, the Red Devils redeemed themselves with a spirited performance which lifted them to the summit of their Champions League group. Here was a Manchester United worthy of the name, a group of players who fought for every yard for the full 90 minutes, and if the circumstances meant forsaking their preferred smooth-passing approach for more direct methods – and leaving Beckham on the bench – the fans were not complaining.

For all that, it was the combative Boavista who made the more thrustful start and Barthez was compelled to make three

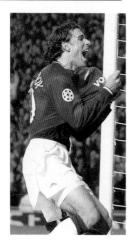

Two more for Ruud van Nistelrooy took his Champions League total to six

0 BOAVISTA

1. RICARDO
23. Nuno Miguel FRECHAUT
25. Armando PETIT
4. PAULO TURRA
5. PEDRO EMANUEL
6. ERIVAN
7. JORGE SILVA
8. DUDA
30. ALEXANDRA GOULART
37. Erwin SANCHEZ
11. SILVA
SUBSTITUTES
2. RUI OSCAR
10. MARCIO SANTOS (11) 58
16. MARTELINHO (7) 61
18. PEDRO SNATOS (37) 69
19. MARIO LOJA
55. GLAUBER
70. Bassey WILLIAM ANDEM

early saves. The first, from Silva, was comfortable, but then a scorcher from Duda demanded an emphatic block and Petit's explosive 30-yarder was tipped over adroitly. Thereafter Scholes, Veron and van Nistelrooy all went close before the mounting tension was eased by a beautifully worked goal, the Dutchman sidefooting home from six yards following a sweet right-flank interchange between Phil Neville and Veron, and a precise cross from the England full-back.

The second half produced an early frightener when Goulart seemed on the point of equalising, only to collide with Silva, thus allowing Gary Neville to scoop clear. But soon the game was effectively decided by two United strikes inside seven minutes. First the unmarked Blanc headed in from a Veron corner, then van Nistelrooy ran on to an exquisite pass from Yorke to clip home his sixth goal of the Champions League campaign.

Now the belief drained visibly from the hitherto feisty Portuguese champions, though they might have grabbed a late consolation had the untended Goulart been more accurate from Martelinho's driven centre.

Overall, the Reds could be immensely proud of a grittily positive reaction to recent adversity.

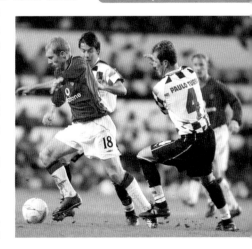

No goals, but a superb contribution from Paul Scholes in midfield helped United put recent travails behind them

MANCHESTER UNITED   0

1. Fabien BARTHEZ
2. Gary NEVILLE
27. Mikael SILVESTRE
16. Roy KEANE
12. Phil NEVILLE
30. John O'SHEA
15. Luke CHADWICK
8. Nicky BUTT
19. Dwight YORKE
20. Ole Gunnar SOLSKJAER
18. Paul SCHOLES

SUBSTITUTES

7. David BECKHAM (15) 59
9. Andy COLE (8) 89
13. Roy CARROLL
22. Ronnie WALLWORK
25. Quinton FORTUNE (19) 82

MATCH REPORT

Manchester United plummeted to their sixth defeat of the League campaign, their third in succession and their first in Premiership history against West Ham. Coming on the back of an apparent renaissance against Boavista, it was a crushing blow to the Red Devils, whose realistic hopes of retaining their title were virtually extinguished by the shock reverse. Driven by the majestic Keane, they worked unstintingly, but their formerly unshakeable confidence and sweet fluency were sadly diminished, so that they were unable to master a doughty, well-organised Hammers side for whom goalkeeper James played magnificently. Yet the hosts began positively, with Keane the inspiration of a sweeping move which ended with Yorke shooting narrowly wide, then Silvestre crashed a ferocious 12-yard drive into the side netting.

Meanwhile, though, Hutchison demanded a sharp save from Barthez with a snap volley and soon it was the Hammers who were looking the more coherent combination. For all that, Scholes might have scored twice before half-time with trademark scorchers, the first set up by Gary Neville and the second by the ubiquitous Keane. On both

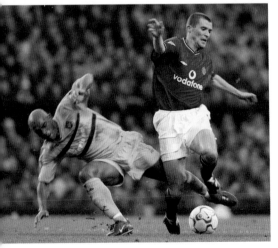

Driven tirelessly by Roy Keane, United were unable to break down their well-organised opponents

1 WEST HAM UNITED

63 DEFOE

1. David JAMES
2. Thomas REPKA
3. Nigel WINTERBURN
4. Don HUTCHISON
30. Sebastien SCHEMMEL
26. Joe COLE
7. Christian DAILLY
8. Trevor SINCLAIR
25. Jermaine DEFOE
10. Paolo DI CANIO
21. Michael CARRICK
SUBSTITUTES
17. Shaka HISLOP
20. Scott MINTO
23. Steve POTTS
28. Laurent COURTOIS
29. Titi CAMARA (25) 84

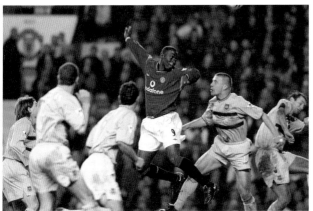

Andy Cole's flying header is admired by the entire West Ham defence, but failed to find the target

occasions the little redhead was foiled by James, who executed a stupendous diving parry followed by a routine stop.

After the interval, the Reds improved and Scholes was unlucky with a glancing header which flashed narrowly wide. But they fell behind to a delightfully crafted goal, instigated by Cole, who eluded several tackles before finding Schemmel on the right. The Frenchman passed inside to Di Canio who swivelled before chipping to the far post, where Defoe headed in. United responded with spirit and might have equalised when a Beckham corner was met by Silvestre's powerful header, only for James to pull off the save of the day. There followed a late siege but, in truth, a breakthrough never looked likely.

MANCHESTER UNITED 5

SOLSKJAER 6, 58
KEANE 10
VAN NISTELROOY 63
SCHOLES 89

1. Fabien BARTHEZ
2. Gary NEVILLE
27. Mikael SILVESTRE
4. Juan Sebastian VERON
30. John O'SHEA
6. Laurent BLANC
16. Roy KEANE
8. Nicky BUTT
20. Ole Gunnar SOLSKJAER
10. Ruud VAN NISTELROOY
18. Paul SCHOLES

SUBSTITUTES

3. Denis IRWIN
7. David BECKHAM
12. Phil NEVILLE
13. Roy CARROLL (1) 83
19. Dwight YORKE (10) 79

MATCH REPORT

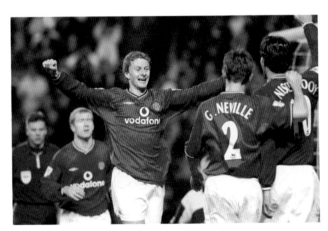

Ole Gunnar Solskjaer is delighted after tapping in his second goal

The Red Devils roared back to form with a devastatingly comprehensive demolition of a Derby County side which never looked remotely capable of challenging the supremacy of their goal-hungry hosts. From the outset, United passed and moved with all their old verve and fluency, and they opened their scoring account with a strike of wondrous quality. Keane found Silvestre on the left and the Frenchman dispatched a low, raking cross which Solskjaer stunned on his chest before netting with a six-yard volley. Four minutes later the tally was doubled after O'Shea broke up a rare Rams raid and stabbed the ball to Keane.

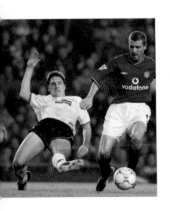

Roy Keane was magnificent once again in the United engine room

0 DERBY COUNTY

24. Andy OAKES
17. Youl MAWENE
16. Luciano ZAVAGNO
38. Francois GRENET
15. Danny HIGGINBOTHAM
6. Chris RIGGOTT
7. Benito CARBONE
37. Pierre DUCROCQ
12. Malcolm CHRISTIE
31. Adam BOLDER
11. Fabrizio RAVANELLI
SUBSTITUTES
9. Deon BURTON (17) 63
10. Giorgi KINKLADZE
21. Adam MURRAY (37) 74
23. Paul BOERTIEN (12) 71
32. Lee GRANT

The ball was ferried to the right flank via Scholes, Keane again and van Nistelrooy, then Solskjaer crossed to the far post where the workaholic skipper popped up to drive home. Thereafter United dominated the remainder of the first period but without adding to the scoreline.

The procession continued after the interval with the Derby keeper deflecting a Scholes volley, then fielding a van Nistelrooy effort before the Dutchman's cross-shot was palmed into the path of Solskjaer, who tapped in. Still United poured forward, though Derby rallied slightly and Barthez made a close-range block from Ravanelli, then repelled a Christie scorcher.

But United, in vivid contrast to recent pallid displays, refused to let up and Butt, Scholes and Keane completed a move of sublime precision which climaxed with van Nistelrooy volleying the fourth goal.

More chances followed for van Nistelrooy and Keane before Scholes got in on the scoring act when he received a pass from the lively Solskjaer, then wrong-footed two defenders before beating Oakes with a fierce low shot.

It was wonderful stuff, but were the Reds just flattering to deceive?

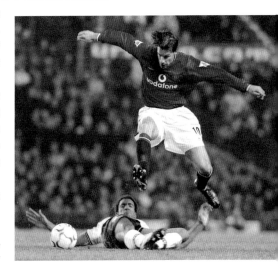

Ruud van Nistelrooy leaps over a grounded Derby defender

MIDDLESBROUGH 0

13. Mark CROSSLEY
27. Robbie STOCKDALE
37. Franck QUEUDREU
12. Jonathon GREENING
17. Ugo EHIOGU
6. Gareth SOUTHGATE
7. Robbie MUSTOE
23. Carlos MARINELLI
9. Paul INCE
19. Hamilton RICARD
11. Alen BOKSIC

SUBSTITUTES

8. Szilard NEMETH
14. Paul OKON
15. Marlon BERESFORD
26. Noel WHELAN (19) 64
28. Colin COOPER

MATCH REPORT

The earlier-than-expected return from injury of Ryan Giggs galvanised the Red Devils into clinching a hard-fought and ultimately deserved victory over former United coach Steve McClaren's doughty but unimaginative Middlesbrough. The inspirational Welshman brought much-needed penetration and balance to the visitors' attack, and within ten minutes of rising from the bench midway through the second half he engineered the decisive strike. Fed by Scholes, he ran at the massed Boro rearguard along the left touchline before squeezing a low centre into the box. Crossley could only palm the ball to the feet of van Nistelrooy, who joyfully netted his 14th goal of the season from five yards.

United, fielding the same outfield ten who had thrashed Derby but with Carroll replacing the unfit Barthez, suffered early disruption with the loss of O'Shea to injury, forcing Gary Neville to move into the middle with brother Phil replacing him at right-back. Not that there was much offensive threat from Boro, who offered no more than three uncharacteristically wan efforts from the energetic Ince during a cagey, incoherent first period, while United were reduced to

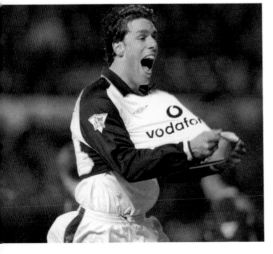

Ruud van Nistelrooy celebrates after scoring his 14th goal of the season

1 MANCHESTER UNITED

76 VAN NISTELROOY

13. Roy CARROLL
2. Gary NEVILLE
27. Mikael SILVESTRE
4. Juan Sebastian VERON
30. John O'SHEA
6. Laurent BLANC
16. Roy KEANE
8. Nicky BUTT
20. Ole Gunnar SOLSKJAER
10. Ruud VAN NISTELROOY
18. Paul SCHOLES
SUBSTITUTES
3. Denis IRWIN
11. Ryan GIGGS (8) 66
12. Phil NEVILLE (30) 13
17. Raimond VAN DER GOUW
19. Dwight YORKE

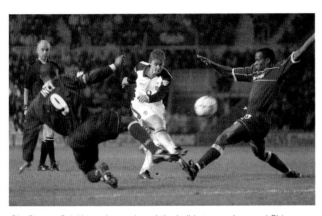

Ole Gunnar Solskjaer tries to thread the ball between Ince and Ehiogu

unconvincing attempts from Solskjaer and van Nistelroy. After the break, though, Sir Alex Ferguson's men showed more thrust and shortly before the hour Butt netted with a far-post header from Keane's cross, only to be penalised for pushing Stockdale.

Now, gradually, the Red Devils established momentum and Silvestre skied from four yards after a Solskjaer corner was flicked on by Keane, then the skipper was through on Crossley only to misdirect his shot. Enter Giggs to fashion the crucial breakthrough, after which he almost scored himself with a snap-volley from 20 yards, only to be foiled by Crossley.

Boro were not buried, though, and they created their two best chances late in the match, when a close-range Whelan volley forced a sharp save from Carroll, then Ince dragged his shot narrowly wide.

MANCHESTER UNITED   6

1. Fabien BARTHEZ
2. Gary NEVILLE
27. Mikael SILVESTRE
4. Juan Sebastian VERON
12. Phil NEVILLE
6. Laurent BLANC
16. Roy KEANE
8. Nicky BUTT
20. Ole Gunnar SOLSKJAER
10. Ruud VAN NISTELROOY
18. Paul SCHOLES

SUBSTITUTES

3. Denis IRWIN
7. David BECKHAM (4) 66
11. Ryan GIGGS (20) 66
13. Roy CARROLL
22. Ronnie WALLWORK (16) 82

VAN NISTELROOY 1, 34, 54
SOLSKJAER 41
KEANE 72
P. NEVILLE 78

MATCH REPORT

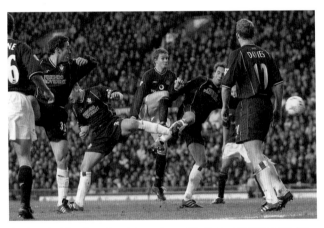

A packed Southampton defence keeps Ole Gunnar Solskjaer out, but was unable to prevent six of the best as United ran rampant

A swashbuckling hat-trick from Ruud van Nistelrooy was the centrepiece of the Red Devils' third successive Premiership victory as they brushed aside Southampton to continue their spirited pursuit of the League leaders. The Dutchman gave a master-class in the centre-forward's art, his deadly finishing matched by his pace and strength, his control and vision, as well as an infectious eagerness for the fray.

But although United dazzled when they poured forward, there was a disturbing tendency for holes to appear at the

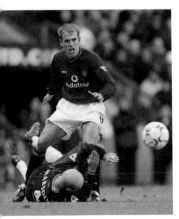

Phil Neville registered his first goal of the season with a 20-yard cracker

1 SOUTHAMPTON

55 PAHARS

1. Paul JONES
2. Jason DODD
3. Wayne BRIDGE
4. Chris MARSDEN
5. Claus LUNDEKVAM
6. Paul WILLIAMS
33. Paul TELFER
12. Anders SVENSSON
9. James BEATTIE
10. Kevin DAVIES
17. Marian PAHARS
SUBSTITUTES
13. Neil MOSS
18. Rory DELAP (12) 81
20. Tahar EL-KHALEJ
24. Dan PETRESCU
36. Brett ORMEROD (10) 59

back as Gordon Strachan's feisty raiders retaliated skilfully. The Reds' start, however, was perfect. Scholes, who went on to display his finest form of the season to date, took possession on the left and drove a majestic 50-yard pass to van Nistelrooy who had slipped free of his marker on the edge of the box. The £19 million man stunned the ball dead with his first touch, then drilled it unerringly past Jones with his second. But Southampton hit back quickly, Telfer heading wide and Beattie dinking marginally high.

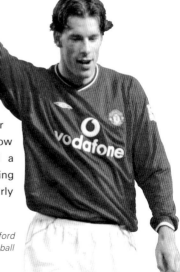

The Reds' attacking rhythm was ever more insistent, though, and they went two ahead when a Solskjaer corner provoked a scramble in which Keane nodded down for van Nistelrooy to bundle in. Next Solskjaer volleyed the third and Giggs' sublime instant through-ball sent in van Nistelrooy to complete his haul with the outside of his right foot before Pahars reduced the arrears. Thereafter Beattie forced two brilliant saves from Barthez but now United were flowing irresistibly, and Keane finished a glorious team move, then Phil Neville climaxed a slaloming run with an unstoppable 20-yarder. Christmas had come early for the Old Trafford faithful.

Hat-trick man Ruud van Nistelrooy walks off the Old Trafford pitch with his reward – the match ball

EVERTON 0

13. Steve SIMONSEN

2. Steve WATSON

15. Gary NAYSMITH

24. Abel XAVIER

5. David WEIR

6. David UNSWORTH

7. Niclas ALEXANDERSSON

8. Tomasz RADZINSKI

16. Thomas GRAVESEN

17. Scot GEMMILL

12. Jesper BLOMQVIST

SUBSTITUTES

1. Paul GERRARD

10. Duncan FERGUSON (12) 73

14. Idan TAL

18. Paul GASCOIGNE (7) 82

19. Joe-Max MOORE

MATCH REPORT

Two gloriously fashioned late goals clinched the Red Devils' 12th triumph in 14 encounters with Everton, an undefeated sequence which extends back to the 1995 FA Cup Final. For the most part this was not a classic contest, with United failing to strike a fluent rhythm until they went ahead, but the telling contributions of Giggs and Beckham, both out of the firing line of late, augured well for continued involvement in the title race. The proceedings might have been more comfortable for the visitors had their predator-in-chief, van Nistelrooy, managed to reach tempting dispatches from Solskjaer and Blanc in the

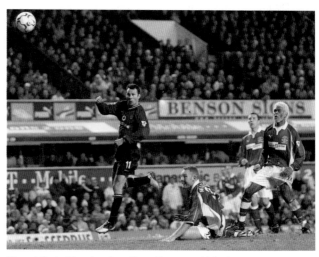

The subtlest of headers from Ryan Giggs puts United one up

2 MANCHESTER UNITED

78 GIGGS
85 VAN NISTELROOY

1. Fabien BARTHEZ
2. Gary NEVILLE
27. Mikael SILVESTRE
4. Juan Sebastian VERON
12. Phil NEVILLE
6. Laurent BLANC
16. Roy KEANE
8. Nicky BUTT
20. Ole Gunnar SOLSKJAER
10. Ruud VAN NISTELROOY
11. Ryan GIGGS
SUBSTITUTES
3. Denis IRWIN
7. David BECKHAM (8) 56
13. Roy CARROLL
19. Dwight YORKE
22. Ronnie WALLWORK

opening minutes, but gradually the hard-working hosts asserted themselves and twice went close to seizing an early advantage. First Barthez leapt salmon-like to repel a Gemmill piledriver, then Unsworth lashed wide from six yards.

United regrouped and forged a handful of openings before the break, Silvestre heading over from Solskjaer's cross, Simonsen saving after the Norwegian had swivelled eight yards out, and van Nistelrooy nodding wide from a Veron centre. At the other end, Moore's deflected overhead kick produced more acrobatics from Barthez.

During the third quarter, there was precious little incident until Beckham arced a fabulous cross from which Giggs netted with a perfect glancing header. The points were made safe when Giggs ran at Naysmith before curling a pass around the Everton rearguard for van Nistelrooy to volley home from six yards. Thereafter the Reds were rampant and Simonsen brought off fine saves to deny Beckham and Keane, but a heavier margin would have been unduly tough on the toiling Toffees.

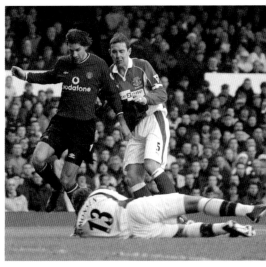

Steve Simonsen, the Everton keeper, dives to save at the feet of Ruud van Nistelrooy

FULHAM 2

1. Edwin VAN DER SAR

2. Steve FINNAN

3. Rufus BREVETT

4. Andy MELVILLE

24. Alain GOMA

14. Steed MALBRANQUE

22. Luis BOA MORTE

18. Sylvain LEGWINSKI

20. Louis SAHA

10. John COLLINS

15. Barry HAYLES

SUBSTITUTES

9. Steve MARLET (15) 89

12. Maik TAYLOR

23. Sean DAVIS (18) 76

25. Abdeslam QUADDOU

40. Andrejs STOLCERS

LEGWINSKI 45
MARLET 89

MATCH REPORT

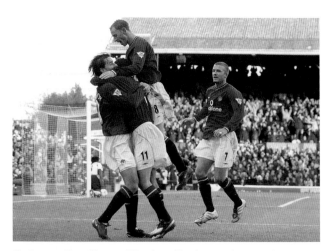

Goalscorers Ryan Giggs and Ruud van Nistelrooy embrace as they put United two goals to the good

Manchester United secured their fifth straight Premiership victory in a five-goal thriller lit up by the incandescent skills of Ryan Giggs. Filling the unaccustomed role of deep-lying strike partner to Ruud van Nistelrooy, the Welshman scored twice with flashes of exquisite opportunism and set up another goal for the Dutchman. Fulham also contributed hugely to the entertainment, netting in the dying minutes to set up a nerve-tingling finale.

The proceedings ignited in the fourth minute when the ball ran loose following a Malbranque corner and Saha volleyed

3 MANCHESTER UNITED

5, 47 GIGGS
45 VAN NISTELROOY

1. Fabien BARTHEZ
2. Gary NEVILLE
27. Mikael SILVESTRE
16. Roy KEANE
12. Phil NEVILLE
6. Laurent BLANC
7. David BECKHAM
8. Nicky BUTT
18. Paul SCHOLES
10. Ruud VAN NISTELROOY
11. Ryan GIGGS
SUBSTITUTES
3. Denis IRWIN
13. Roy CARROLL
19. Dwight YORKE
20. Ole Gunnar SOLSKJAER
22. Ronnie WALLWORK

against the bar from 12 yards. It was a lucky escape and United capitalised ruthlessly by taking the lead within a minute, van der Sar miskicking a lofted through-pass from Scholes, Giggs coolly threading into the empty net from 25 yards. An interlude of end-to-end action ensued, with van der Sar blocking an acute-angled volley from van Nistelrooy and Blanc's header from a Giggs corner, then Hayles' shot cannoned off United's bar and Barthez saved the follow-up from Malbranque.

There was barely time to draw breath before the Reds' keeper was tipping over Malbranque's 28-yard free-kick, Blanc was heading wide from another Giggs dispatch and van der Sar was frustrating Butt and Scholes from close range.

More goals seemed inevitable and three came in two minutes either side of the break. First van Nistelrooy volleyed home from six yards after a slick one-two with Giggs, then the unmarked Legwinski headed in from a free-kick, only for Giggs to net with a fabulous half-volley from the corner of the six-yard box.

Thereafter United took control until Brevett weaved down the Fulham left and crossed for Marlet to tap in, causing late palpitations in the visitors' camp.

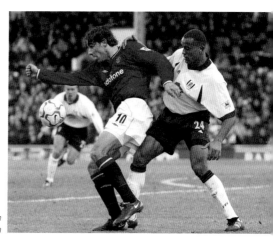

Ruud van Nistelrooy shields the ball from Fulham's Alain Goma

DECEMBER IN REVIEW

SATURDAY 1	v CHELSEA	H	0-3
WEDNESDAY 5	v BOAVISTA	H	3-0
SATURDAY 8	v WEST HAM UNITED	H	0-1
WEDNESDAY 12	v DERBY COUNTY	H	5-0
SATURDAY 15	v MIDDLESBROUGH	A	1-0
SATURDAY 22	v SOUTHAMPTON	H	6-1
WEDNESDAY 26	v EVERTON	A	2-0
SUNDAY 30	v FULHAM	A	3-2

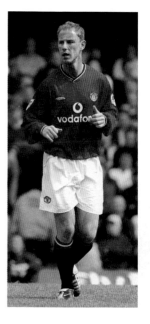

PLAYER IN THE FRAME

Nicky Butt

Never the most flamboyant of performers, Nicky can take enormous credit for his part in reviving United's fortunes after a dismal autumn. He contributed mightily to a crucial victory against Boavista, and then emerged as a key figure in the lengthy winning run which followed, displaying more skill than many pundits credit him with possessing.

FA BARCLAYCARD PREMIERSHIP

UP TO AND INCLUDING
THURSDAY 27 DECEMBER 2001

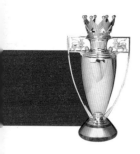

	P	W	D	L	F	A	Pts
Newcastle United	19	12	3	4	37	23	39
Arsenal	19	10	6	3	39	23	36
Liverpool	18	11	3	4	28	18	36
Leeds United	19	9	8	2	29	17	35
MANCHESTER UNITED	19	10	3	6	45	28	33
Chelsea	19	7	9	3	29	15	30
Tottenham Hotspur	19	8	3	8	30	26	27
Aston Villa	19	7	6	6	25	24	27
Sunderland	19	7	5	7	17	17	26
Fulham	18	5	9	4	17	17	24
West Ham United	19	6	6	7	24	30	24
Charlton Athletic	19	5	8	6	21	22	23
Everton	19	6	5	8	23	25	23
Blackburn Rovers	19	5	7	7	25	24	22
Bolton Wanderers	19	5	6	8	21	29	21
Middlesbrough	18	5	4	9	17	26	19
Southampton	18	6	1	11	19	30	19
Derby County	19	4	4	11	14	35	16
Ipswich Town	19	3	6	10	19	28	15
Leicester City	19	3	6	10	12	34	15

JANUARY

WEDNESDAY 2	v NEWCASTLE UNITED	H
SUNDAY 6	v ASTON VILLA	A
SUNDAY 13	v SOUTHAMPTON	A
SATURDAY 19	v BLACKBURN ROVERS	H
TUESDAY 22	v LIVERPOOL	H
SATURDAY 26	v MIDDLESBROUGH	A
TUESDAY 29	v BOLTON WANDERERS	A

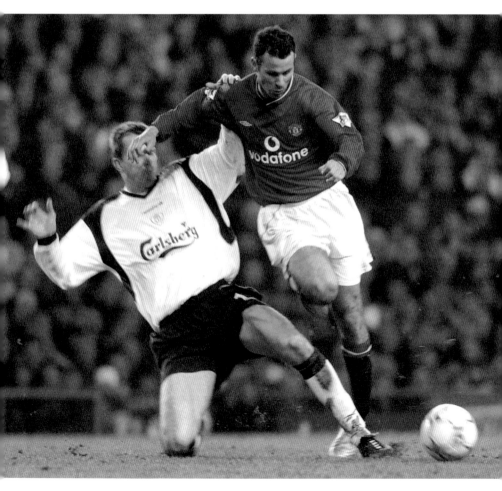

MANCHESTER UNITED 3

VAN NISTELROOY 24
SCHOLES 50, 62

1. Fabien BARTHEZ
2. Gary NEVILLE
27. Mikael SILVESTRE
4. Juan Sebastian VERON
12. Phil NEVILLE
6. Laurent BLANC
16. Roy KEANE
8. Nicky BUTT
20. Ole Gunnar SOLSKJAER
10. Ruud VAN NISTELROOY
18. Paul SCHOLES

SUBSTITUTES

3. Denis IRWIN
7. David BECKHAM (20) 85
13. Roy CARROLL
19. Dwight YORKE (10) 66
30. John O'SHEA

MATCH REPORT

The Red Devils' revival continued to gather momentum with a sixth consecutive League win. Though the performance was by no means one of United's best, they scintillated at times, particularly with their passing and movement. However, unusually for visitors to Old Trafford, it was Newcastle who enjoyed the lion's share of possession and it was they who had the first chance after eight minutes, when Speed's crisp volley following a corner was headed off the line by Phil Neville.

Seven in a row: Ruud van Nistelrooy heads home from Mikael Silvestre's cross to score in his seventh consecutive match

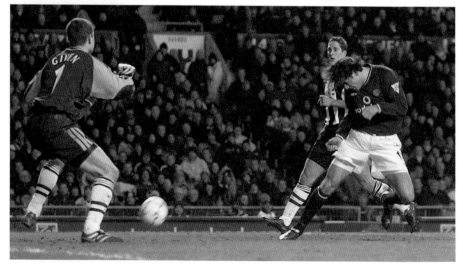

1 NEWCASTLE UNITED

69 SHEARER

1. Shay GIVEN
18. Aaron HUGHES
3. Robbie ELLIOT
4. Nolberto SOLANO
34. Nikolas DABIZAS
24. Sylvain DISTIN
7. Robert LEE
8. Kieron DYER
9. Alan SHEARER
17. Craig BELLAMY
11. Gary SPEED
SUBSTITUTES
5. Andrew O'BRIEN
13. Steve HARPER
20. Lomana LUALUA
23. Shola AMEOBI (4) 81
35. Olvier BERNARD (17) 81

The Reds replied with a rampaging run and explosive shot from van Nistelrooy, which Given diverted for a corner, and it was the Dutchman, scoring in his seventh successive senior outing, who gave them the lead. Butt found Solskjaer on the left, Silvestre overlapped and the Frenchman's cross allowed the untended marksman to head in from five yards. But Newcastle rallied, Elliott was allowed too much freedom on the left and, from one of his crosses on 42 minutes, Solano nodded past Barthez, only for the strike to be ruled out for a push on Silvestre.

Soon after the break United scored again when Butt's pass reached Silvestre on the left, the ball was switched inside to Solskjaer, then to Scholes, who swivelled to net from 14 yards. Solano and Bellamy threatened instant reprisal, but failed to register and paid the price when Solskjaer slipped the ball to Keane, who surged into the Geordies' box and crossed to Scholes, who converted deftly at the far post.

Still Bobby Robson's battlers refused to yield and after Shearer reduced the arrears with a magnificent header from yet another Elliott centre, a tremor of anxiety rippled around Old Trafford. The Reds were never really stretched again, however, and twice Solskjaer almost extended the victory margin.

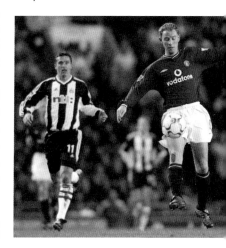

Nicky Butt worked hard in midfield all evening and had a hand in two of United's goals

ASTON VILLA 2

1. Peter SCHMEICHEL
31. Jlloyd SAMUEL
3. Alan WRIGHT
4. Olof MELLBERG
17. Lee HENDRIE
6. George BOATENG
7. Ian TAYLOR
8. Juan Pablo ANGEL
22. Darius VASSELL
10. Paul MERSON
11. Steve STAUNTON

SUBSTITUTES

2. Mark DELANEY
12. Peter ENCKELMAN
15. Gareth BARRY (6) 86
18. Steve STONE (3) 86
20. Moustapha HADJI (10) 86

TAYLOR 52
P. NEVILLE (o.g.) 54

MATCH REPORT

Stunning comebacks have become a Manchester United speciality, but even they have rarely turned a contest on its head in quite such a devastating and dramatic fashion. Two down, albeit against the run of play, and with time running out, Sir Alex Ferguson's miracle-workers plundered three goals in the space of six pulsating minutes to transform what had been merely a fascinating encounter into an FA Cup classic. At the core of the Reds' remarkable resurgence was Ruud van Nistelrooy, who rose from the bench to supply two fabulous strikes, underlining vividly his burgeoning stature as a world-class marksman.

The first half had been a curious affair, with United stroking the ball around fluently but being largely frustrated by a well-organised Villa side content to soak up pressure and, perhaps, snatch an advantage on the break. Schmeichel dealt comfortably with firm efforts by Beckham and Solskjaer, while the Norwegian and Chadwick (twice) were inaccurate when well placed. For their part, Villa could not muster a single shot on target during the opening period.

After the break United looked ever-more dominant before the hosts seemed to take control with two goals in two minutes. First Taylor latched on to a

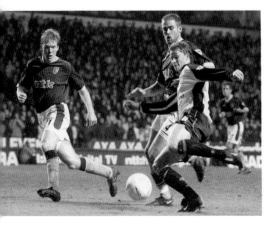

Ole Gunnar Solskjaer swivels to despatch a half-volley into the Villa net to start United's comeback

3 MANCHESTER UNITED

77 SOLSKJAER
80, 82 VAN NISTELROOY

13. Roy CARROLL

2. Gary NEVILLE

27. Mikael SILVESTRE

4. Juan Sebastian VERON

12. Phil NEVILLE

6. Laurent BLANC

7. David BECKHAM

8. Nicky BUTT

20. Ole Gunnar SOLSKJAER

16. Roy KEANE

18. Paul SCHOLES

SUBSTITUTES

10. Ruud VAN NISTELROOY (15) 56

15. Luke CHADWICK (8) 26

17. Raimond VAN DER GOUW

28. Michael STEWART

30. John O'SHEA

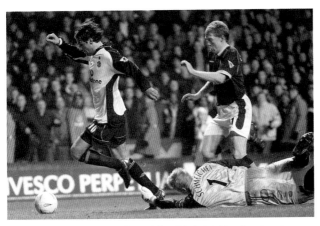

Ruud van Nistelrooy leaves Peter Schmeichel clutching the air as he rounds the keeper before netting United's dramatic late winner

Hendrie through-pass before toe-poking inside a post from 14 yards, then poor Phil Neville nodded past the wrong-footed Carroll. Villa held on for 23 minutes before the storm broke when Solskjaer accepted a dispatch from Silvestre, swivelled brilliantly past Mellberg and netted with a stinging half-volley.

Three minutes later Scholes chipped to the far post, Beckham nodded down and van Nistelrooy stunned the ball on his chest, then volleyed thunderously into the roof of the net. Now United were unstoppable and they broke Villa's hearts when Solskjaer slid the ball to van Nistelrooy, who rounded Schmeichel and netted imperiously to provide a fitting climax to an unforgettable match.

SOUTHAMPTON 1

BEATTIE 3

1. Paul JONES
2. Jason DODD
3. Wayne BRIDGE
4. Chris MARSDEN
5. Claus LUNDEKVAM
6. Paul WILLIAMS
33. Paul TELFER
12. Anders SVENSSON
9. James BEATTIE
29. Fabrice FERNANDES
17. Marian PAHARS

SUBSTITUTES

13. Neil MOSS
24. Dan PETRESCU
25. Gary MONK
34. Agustin DELGADO (9) 26
36. Brett ORMEROD (29) 60

MATCH REPORT

Manchester United scaled the Premiership summit for the first time during the season thanks to a seventh successive League win, all of which had featured at least one goal by Ruud van Nistelrooy, who thus equalled the competition record for scoring in consecutive games. However, this was no mere routine victory against an accomplished Southampton side who seized an early lead, then twice rapped the frame of the Red Devils' goal when the scores were level. United had not completed their first three minutes of football at St Mary's when they fell a goal behind after Silvestre conceded possession, Dodd crossed from the right and Beattie brushed aside Blanc to net with an emphatic downward header from 12 yards.

An attractively open contest developed and soon the visitors levelled in majestic manner. Gary Neville found Beckham with a raking pass, then van Nistelrooy flicked to Scholes and the England midfielder supplied an instant return delivery, allowing the rampant Dutchman to charge into the box and shoot past Jones from a narrow angle.

The Saints reacted positively and were unlucky not to regain their lead after 32 minutes when Delgado headed against a post, then again nine minutes later when the enterprising substitute set up Pahars, whose shot clipped the bar instead of bulging a gaping net. So it was against the run of play when Beckham's unerringly curled 25-yard free-kick gave the Reds an interval

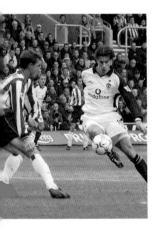

Ruud van Nistelrooy flicks the ball forward. An instant return from Paul Scholes allowed the Dutchman to score United's equaliser

3 MANCHESTER UNITED

9 VAN NISTELROOY
45 BECKHAM
63 SOLSKJAER

1. Fabien BARTHEZ
2. Gary NEVILLE
27. Mikael SILVESTRE
4. Juan Sebastian VERON
12. Phil NEVILLE
6. Laurent BLANC
7. David BECKHAM
16. Roy KEANE
20. Ole Gunnar SOLSKJAER
10. Ruud VAN NISTELROOY
18. Paul SCHOLES
SUBSTITUTES
3. Denis IRWIN (12) h-t
11. Ryan GIGGS (10) 85
13. Roy CARROLL
15. Luke CHADWICK
28. Michael STEWART

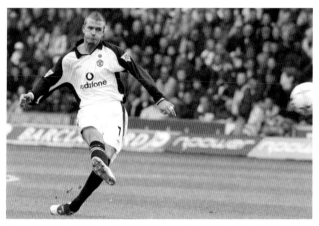

Seconds before half time, David Beckham curled a 25-yard free-kick past Saints' keeper Paul Jones to give United the lead

advantage, one which he almost increased with another set piece immediately after the break, only to be foiled by Jones.

Thereafter the action ebbed and flowed until United's decisive third strike, set up by van Nistelrooy and executed fiercely from 16 yards by Solskjaer. Later the dangerous Delgado went close with a bicycle kick and a header, which brought a brilliant save from Barthez, but by then the destination of the points was pretty well sealed.

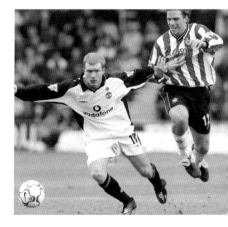

Paul Scholes sidesteps Southampton's Anders Svennson during a combative midfield tussle

MANCHESTER UNITED 2

VAN NISTELROOY (pen.) 45
KEANE 81

1. Fabien BARTHEZ
2. Gary NEVILLE
27. Mikael SILVESTRE
4. Juan Sebastian VERON
12. Phil NEVILLE
6. Laurent BLANC
7. David BECKHAM
16. Roy KEANE
20. Ole Gunnar SOLSKJAER
10. Ruud VAN NISTELROOY
18. Paul SCHOLES

SUBSTITUTES

3. Denis IRWIN (27) h-t
8. Nicky BUTT (4) 84
11. Ryan GIGGS (20) 56
13. Roy CARROLL
30. John O'SHEA

MATCH REPORT

The Red Devils were a trifle fortunate to claim all three points on a day of tumbling records at Old Trafford. Ruud van Nistelrooy became the first man to score in eight consecutive Premiership games, United chalked up a century of League matches without a 0-0 draw and Sir Alex Ferguson announced an unchanged side for the first time in 97 contests. More importantly, though, victory saw the Reds move two points clear at the top of the table.

The match began with Cole – how peculiar to see him in blue-and-white halves – almost setting up Jansen, only for an alert Barthez to neutralise the threat. Neill cleared off his line from Solskjaer, and Scholes executed a glorious one-two with Veron before shaving an upright with a powerful 20-yarder, but Blackburn were playing well, too, and Jansen shot straight at

Laurent Blanc is felled in the penalty area by the Blackburn defence...

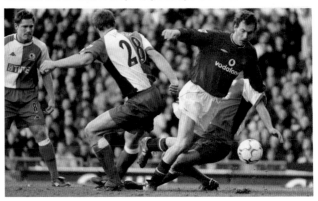

1 BLACKBURN ROVERS

49 HIGNETT

1. Brad FRIEDEL
31. Lucas NEILL
3. TUGAY Kerimoglu
28. Martin TAYLOR
5. Stig Inge BJORNEBYE
6. Nils-Eric JOHANSSON
15. Craig HIGNETT
8. David DUNNE
9. Andy COLE
10. Matt JANSEN
11. Damien DUFF
SUBSTITUTES
4. Henning BERG
7. Garry FLITCROFT (8) 65
12. Mark HUGHES (10) 73
21. Corrado GRABBI (5) 84
23. Alan KELLY

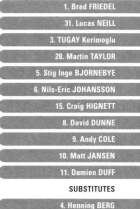

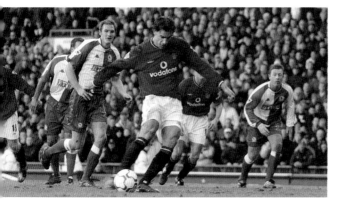

... and Ruud van Nistelrooy scores from the resultant penalty. Goals in eight consecutive matches gave him a new Premiership record

Barthez, and Silvestre blocked Hignett at the far post. The Reds took the lead in first-half stoppage time when Blanc waltzed past two defenders before apparently being floored by Friedel, and van Nistelrooy crashed home from the spot to make history.

Almost immediately after the break Rovers retaliated when Jansen sent in Hignett who scored from eight yards. Soon they might have gone ahead when Tugay freed Duff, only for Barthez to block his shot, then at the other end van Nistelrooy shivered the bar with a bicycle kick following Veron's sublime chip.

The decisive strike came from Keane following great work by Scholes and a lovely Giggs backheel, but still there was time for Flitcroft and Neill to go close for the irrepressible visitors.

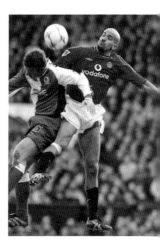

Juan Sebastian Veron tussles for possession with Blackburn's Bjornebye

MANCHESTER UNITED 0

1. Fabien BARTHEZ
2. Gary NEVILLE
27. Mikael SILVESTRE
4. Juan Sebastian VERON
12. Phil NEVILLE
6. Laurent BLANC
7. David BECKHAM
16. Roy KEANE
18. Paul SCHOLES
10. Ruud VAN NISTELROOY
11. Ryan GIGGS

SUBSTITUTES

8. Nicky BUTT
13. Roy CARROLL
20. Ole Gunnar SOLSKJAER (7) 88
22. Ronnie WALLWORK
30. John O'SHEA

MATCH REPORT

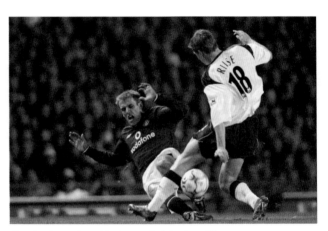

Phil Neville tangles with Liverpool's John Arne Riise

The Red Devils' victorious run came to a traumatic end, as did the recent phenomenal scoring sequence of Ruud van Nistelrooy, as Liverpool mocked the form-book to record their fifth straight victory over their fiercest rivals. It was a frustrating night for United, who started confidently and dominated for the opening 30 minutes. But then, slowly but inexorably, the cautious Merseysiders asserted themselves and it was they who played the most coherent football in the second half.

Despite their initial superiority, Sir Alex Ferguson's men found it difficult to engineer scoring opportunities and the first clear chance did not materialise until the 16th minute when

1 LIVERPOOL

85 MURPHY

12. Jerzy DUDEK
2. Stephane HENCHOZ
23. Jamie CARRAGHER
4. Sami HYYPIA
29. Stephen WRIGHT
16. Dietmar HAMANN
17. Steven GERRARD
8. Emile HESKEY
13. Danny MURPHY
10. Michael OWEN
18. John Arne RIISE

SUBSTITUTES

9. Nicolas ANELKA (10) 77
15. Patrik BERGER (13) 88
19. Pegguy ARPHEXAD
21. Gary McALLISTER
25. Igor BISCAN

Silvestre's driven cross was half-cleared to Giggs, who drilled a low shot just beyond Dudek's far post. Then, as United counter-attacked rapidly following a rare Liverpool corner, Scholes fired a dipping 20-yarder fractionally wide.

Further pressure was applied but Veron was off target from 20 yards, Giggs combined neatly with Scholes only for Henchoz to deflect his shot, then the Swiss defender, who policed van Nistelrooy admirably all evening, twice foiled the Dutchman. In retaliation Owen drove wide from 25 yards, but it was the hosts who ended the first period on the front foot, with van Nistelrooy just failing to reach a fizzing cross from Scholes.

The second half saw Liverpool grow in stature, gradually gaining midfield ascendancy, and it was not until the 73rd minute that Dudek was tested again, when he parried a Veron scorcher.

At the other end, Anelka's close-range volley brought a brilliant block from Barthez, who then repelled Riise's 25-yarder, but the Frenchman was helpless a prevent the late winner, a delicate six-yard dink from Murphy, who had been fed superbly by Gerrard. Almost immediately a Giggs header from a Silvestre cross brought a diving save from Dudek, but after that Liverpool survived a belated series of attacks with relative ease.

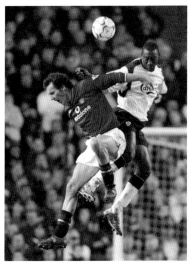

Laurent Blanc is helpless to prevent Emily Heskey heading into the United box

MIDDLESBROUGH 2

WHELAN 85
CAMPBELL 89

13. Mark CROSSLEY
27. Robbie STOCKDALE
37. Franck QUEUDREU
12. Jonathon GREENING
28. Colin COOPER
6. Gareth SOUTHGATE
7. Robbie MUSTOE
23. Carlos MARINELLI
26. Noel WHELAN
20. Dean WINDASS
32. Allan JOHNSTON

SUBSTITUTES

15. Marlon BERESFORD
18. Andy CAMPBELL (21) 75
19. Hamilton RICARD
21. Mark WILSON (23) h-t
29. Jason GAVIN (32) h-t

MATCH REPORT

A calamitous late error of judgement by Laurent Blanc precipitated the Red Devils' shock exit from the FA Cup at the hands of their former coach, Steve McClaren.

It was particularly galling as the blunder, which ended a run of imperious form from the classy veteran, occurred late in a contest during which United had bossed the first half comprehensively, then spurned several clear-cut openings in the second. A routine clearance was in prospect as Crossley's long downfield punt seemed to be dropping comfortably on to the

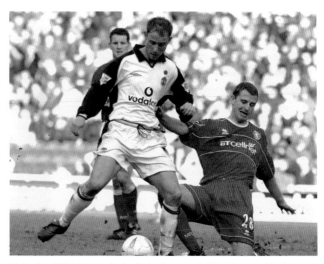

United's midfield, in particular Nicky Butt, worked hard to provide the stikers with chances – but they were unable to take them

0 MANCHESTER UNITED

1. Fabien BARTHEZ
2. Gary NEVILLE
27. Mikael SILVESTRE
22. Ronnie WALLWORK
12. Phil NEVILLE
6. Laurent BLANC
15. Luke CHADWICK
8. Nicky BUTT
20. Ole Gunnar SOLSKJAER
16. Roy KEANE
18. Paul SCHOLES

SUBSTITUTES

10. Ruud VAN NISTELROOY (15) 61
11. Ryan GIGGS (22) 61
13. Roy CARROLL
19. Dwight YORKE (20) 80
30. John O'SHEA

Frenchman's head, but he let it sail behind him, allowing Whelan to nip in and poke the ball under Barthez from six yards. Then, with the visitors committed to all-out attack in search of an equaliser, Boro seized on a weak kick by the goalkeeper, Whelan found Windass on the right and the subsequent centre was headed home by the untended Campbell.

No one who had witnessed the one-way first period could have predicted such an outcome. After Keane had clipped the hosts' near post with a first-minute cross, Mustoe headed a Wallwork header off his goal-line with Crossley beaten, and Butt, Scholes and Solskjaer were all off target when favourably placed. Boro had been toothless to that point, but McClaren switched formation to 3-5-2 at the interval and his side was transformed, with Wilson, Stockdale and Windass all bringing saves from Barthez within six minutes of the restart.

United then introduced Giggs and van Nistelrooy in a bid to force the issue. For one fleeting moment, as Silvestre met a corner with a thunderous header, the ploy looked to have paid rich dividends, only for Mustoe to pull off another goal-line clearance. More pressure from the visitors ensued, but a no-score draw seemed likely … and then came that demoralising denouement.

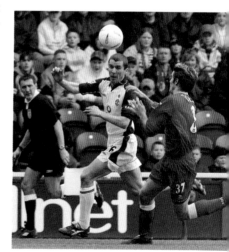

Roy Keane shows off his close control as he gallops past Boro defender Franck Queudreu

BOLTON WANDERERS 0

22. Jussi JAASKELAINEN

20. Nicky SOUTHALL

3. Mike WHITLOW

4. Gudni BERGSSON

24. Anthony BARNESS

14. Gareth FARRELLY

7. Bo HANSEN

15. Kevin NOLAN

17. Michael RICKETTS

16. Fredi BOBIC

11. Ricardo GARDNER

SUBSTITUTES

9. Henrik PEDERSEN

10. Dean HOLDSWORTH (16) 75

25. Simon CHARLTON (2) h-t

28 Jermaine JOHNSON (7) 59

30. Kevin POOLE

MATCH REPORT

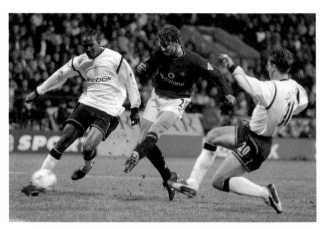

Ole Gunnar Solskjaer nips between two defenders to sidefoot United into a 15th-minute lead

A superlative Ole Gunnar Solskjaer hat-trick and two stupendous saves by Fabien Barthez were the centrepieces of a majestic display by Manchester United. Smarting from back-to-back defeats, Sir Alex Ferguson called for his men to lift themselves into overdrive. But although the Red Devils richly deserved their win, it should be pointed out that a spirited Bolton side fashioned plenty of chances of their own.

Indeed, the Trotters began at an impressive gallop, with Bobic and Ricketts going close in the first seven minutes, only to be halted in their tracks by a classic United counter-attack. Van

4 MANCHESTER UNITED

15, 39, 64 SOLSKJAER
83 VAN NISTELROOY

1. Fabien BARTHEZ
2. Gary NEVILLE
27. Mikael SILVESTRE
16. Roy KEANE
12. Phil NEVILLE
6. Laurent BLANC
7. David BECKHAM
18. Paul SCHOLES
20. Ole Gunnar SOLSKJAER
10. Ruud VAN NISTELROOY
11. Ryan GIGGS

8. Nicky BUTT (16) 73
13. Roy CARROLL
21. Diego FORLAN (20) 76
24. Wesley BROWN
30. John O'SHEA (6) 72

Nistelrooy won the ball deep inside his own half and fed Giggs with an exquisite pass. The Welshman lacerated the Bolton rearguard with his pace before squaring for Solskjaer to net clinically from 12 yards. Now the visitors assumed command, passing deliciously, before Solskjaer doubled the lead with an adroit near-post header from Beckham's corner.

Shortly before the break Bolton might have retaliated but the flying Barthez parried a powerful Ricketts volley, then within seconds of the restart United almost grabbed a third when Giggs shot against a post and Beckham skied the rebound.

After 54 minutes Barthez made another brilliant save, this time from a Ricketts header, but soon the Reds moved out of Bolton's reach when Solskjaer completed his hat-trick with a deft, stooping nod from a Beckham free-kick.

Though United were now in cruise control, further openings were fashioned at either end, only one of which was taken. That fell to van Nistelroy, who started a lovely move which flowed on through Beckham and Giggs before the Dutchman was presented with the formality of a six-yard tap-in.

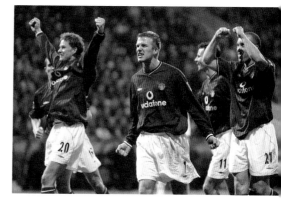

Ole Gunnar Solskjaer salutes the travelling United fans. Roy Keane, David Beckham, Ryan Giggs and Mikael Silvestre join the party

January in Review

WEDNESDAY 2	v NEWCASTLE UNITED	H	3-1
SUNDAY 6	v ASTON VILLA	A	3-2
SUNDAY 13	v SOUTHAMPTON	A	3-1
SATURDAY 19	v BLACKBURN ROVERS	H	2-1
TUESDAY 22	v LIVERPOOL	H	0-1
SATURDAY 26	v MIDDLESBROUGH	A	0-2
TUESDAY 29	v BOLTON WANDERERS	A	4-0

PLAYER IN THE FRAME

Gary Neville

The England stalwart was at his ultra-reliable best as the Red Devils sought to consolidate their improved form in the New Year. He settled into a stable central defensive partnership with Laurent Blanc, allowing brother Phil to enjoy an impressive stint at right-back. Gary was the rock upon which Newcastle, Southampton, Blackburn and Bolton all foundered.

FA Barclaycard Premiership

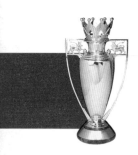

	P	W	D	L	F	A	Pts
MANCHESTER UNITED	25	15	3	7	60	34	48
Arsenal	24	13	8	3	49	29	47
Newcastle United	24	14	4	6	45	30	46
Liverpool	25	13	7	5	34	24	46
Leeds United	24	11	9	4	35	23	42
Chelsea	24	10	10	4	42	23	40
Aston Villa	24	9	9	6	31	28	36
Tottenham Hotspur	24	9	5	10	35	33	32
Charlton Athletic	24	8	8	8	30	30	32
Fulham	23	7	10	6	23	23	31
Southampton	24	9	2	13	29	37	29
Everton	24	7	7	10	25	30	28
Sunderland	24	7	7	10	19	26	28
West Ham United	24	7	7	10	27	41	28
Ipswich Town	24	7	6	11	32	33	27
Middlesbrough	23	7	5	11	22	31	26
Blackburn Rovers	24	6	7	11	32	32	25
Bolton Wanderers	24	5	10	9	27	39	25
Derby County	24	5	4	15	17	42	19
Leicester City	24	3	8	13	15	41	17

UP TO AND INCLUDING
WEDNESDAY 31 JANUARY 2002

FEBRUARY

SATURDAY 2	v SUNDERLAND	H
SUNDAY 10	v CHARLTON ATHLETIC	A
WEDNESDAY 20	v NANTES ATLANTIQUE	A
SATURDAY 23	v ASTON VILLA	H
TUESDAY 26	v NANTES ATLANTIQUE	H

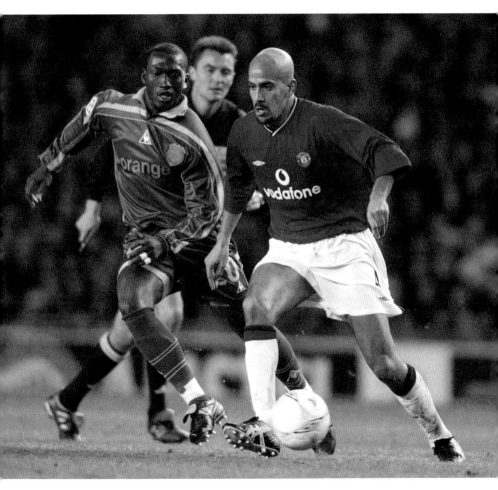

FA BARCLAYCARD PREMIERSHIP
Saturday 2 February, 2002

MANCHESTER UNITED 4

1. Fabien BARTHEZ
2. Gary NEVILLE
27. Mikael SILVESTRE
16. Roy KEANE
12. Phil NEVILLE
6. Laurent BLANC
7. David BECKHAM
18. Paul SCHOLES
20. Ole Gunnar SOLSKJAER
10. Ruud VAN NISTELROOY
11. Ryan GIGGS

SUBSTITUTES

3. Denis IRWIN
8. Nicky BUTT (16) 79
13. Roy CARROLL
21. Diego FORLAN (11) 64
30. John O'SHEA (6) 64

P. NEVILLE 6
BECKHAM 25
VAN NISTELROOY 28, 44 (pen.)

MATCH REPORT

The Red Devils scalded the Black Cats with an irresistible first-half display of compelling brilliance. With Giggs and Beckham at their most devastating, United attacked fluently from the first whistle, and there never seemed the remotest prospect of the visitors securing their first Old Trafford victory for 34 years.

The opening goal offered an apt summation of the one-sided contest, with a 13-pass move purring towards a climax via Beckham and van Nistelrooy before Solskjaer's defence-splitting dispatch freed the charging Philip Neville to net with a cross-shot from six yards. True, Sunderland quickly found themselves on level terms when Phillips was allowed to turn and surprise Barthez with a low 30-yarder, but United's response was merciless. Undeterred by the spongy surface, they popped the ball around with crisp accuracy, creating chance after chance. Silvestre was off target with a free header and Solskjaer failed to turn home from one yard out, then Beckham capped a sinuous run with a 25-yard curler which brought the best from Macho.

So much for the misses; soon the hits began. After Beckham had restored the lead with a copybook free-kick, van Nistelrooy contributed the goal of the day, perhaps of the season. The England captain played the ball into the Dutchman, whose first touch took him to the side

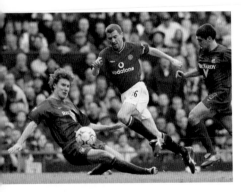

Roy Keane powers his way between Varga and Reyna to set up yet another chance for United's strikers

1 SUNDERLAND

12 PHILLIPS

30. Jurgen MACHO
2. Bernt HAAS
3. Michael GRAY
4. Claudio REYNA
5. Stanislav VARGA
17. Jody CRADDOCK
16. Jason McATEER
18. Darren WILLIAMS
12. Joachim BJORKLUND
10. Kevin PHILLIPS
11. Kevin KILBANE
SUBSTITUTES
9. Niall QUINN (16) 61
13. Michael INGHAM
15. David BELLION
24. George McCARTNEY (2) 61
33. Julio ARCA (5) h-t

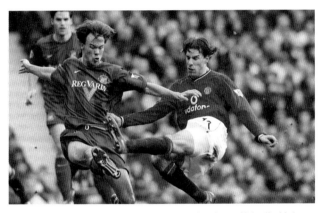

Goal of the Season? Ruud van Nistelrooy crashes home United's third

of Bjorkland before he swivelled to unleash a thunderous left-foot volley past Macho from 12 yards. With the Reds ever more rampant, a scintillating Silvestre surge set up Giggs, who was denied by Macho, then Solskjaer and Beckham nearly added to the tally before Giggs was impeded by Varga and van Nistelrooy converted from the spot.

Unsurprisingly United cruised through the second period, the only incidents being flying parries by Barthez from Phillips at one end and Macho from Scholes at the other. But by then, it was all academic.

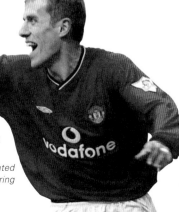

Phil Neville looks suitably delighted after opening the scoring

CHARLTON ATHLETIC 0

1. Dean KIELY
19. Luke YOUNG
3. Chris POWELL
4. Graham STUART
36. Mark FISH
27. Jorge COSTA
7. Chris BART-WILLIAMS
29. Kevin LISBIE
9. Jason EUELL
17. Scott PARKER
11. John ROBINSON

SUBSTITUTES

13. Sasa ILIC
18. Paul KONCHESKY (29) 82
21. Jonatan JOHANSSON (9) 82
24. Jon FORTUNE
26. Mathias SVENSSON (4) 73

MATCH REPORT

A brilliant brace by arch-opportunist Ole Gunnar Solskjaer lifted the Red Devils back to the Premiership summit. Both his goals were poached with exquisite touch and timing as he continued to display the most compelling form of his career.

It should be stressed, though, that United never had it all their own way against the feisty Addicks, who justified their position in the top half of the table and pushed forward enterprisingly for much of the match.

Certainly Charlton began brightly, pinning their visitors back, though they failed to create scoring chances while Sir Alex Ferguson's men menaced on a series of slick counter-attacks.

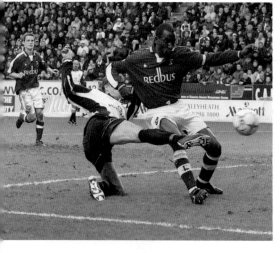

From one of these Giggs fired wide and from another Keane brought a fine diving save from Kiely, then Beckham's volley was deflected to safety.

The breakthrough was as simple as it was utterly devastating. Keane played a glorious 60-yard diagonal pass to Solskjaer, who eluded Fish and took the plummeting ball deliciously in his stride before curling home a waspish cross-shot from 12 yards. At the other end a loose header from Silvestre precipitated a scramble in which Carroll saved

Ole Gunnar Solskjaer wraps his foot around Chris Powell to secure the points for United...

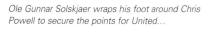

2 MANCHESTER UNITED

33, 74 SOLSKJAER

13. Roy CARROLL
2. Gary NEVILLE
27. Mikael SILVESTRE
16. Roy KEANE
12. Phil NEVILLE
6. Laurent BLANC
7. David BECKHAM
18. Paul SCHOLES
20. Ole Gunnar SOLSKJAER
10. Ruud VAN NISTELROOY
11. Ryan GIGGS
SUBSTITUTES
3. Denis IRWIN
4. Juan Sebastian VERON (10) 67
8. Nicky BUTT (11) 88
17. Raimond VAN DER GOUW
21. Diego FORLAN (20) 78

desperately at Euell's feet, then, in first-half stoppage time, Bart-Williams was wide with Charlton's first shot.

After the break Solskjaer twice went close before Euell missed a golden opportunity to level by heading wide from close range after Fish had nodded on a Bart-Williams corner. Ten minutes later Stuart thought he had equalised from three yards only to be ruled offside, but soon the issue was effectively settled in devastating style. Keane found Beckham on the right and the England captain crossed to Giggs, whose shot on the turn was parried admirably by Kiely. It seemed that Powell had the danger covered only for Solskjaer to snake out a foot and convert deftly from a narrow angle. It was yet another heavenly addition to the Norwegian's princely portfolio of goals.

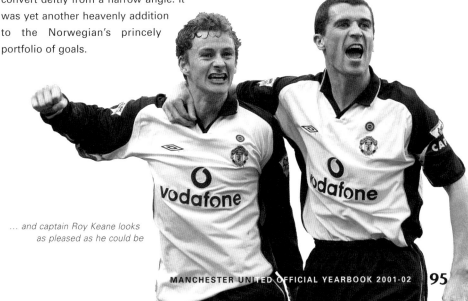

… and captain Roy Keane looks as pleased as he could be

Nantes Atlantique 1

MOLDOVAN 9

1. Mickaël LANDREAU
2. Nestor FABBRI
19. Marama VAHIRUA
4. Mario YEPES
22. Sylvain ARMAND
6. Mathieu BERSON
35. Mauro CETTO
21. Olivier QUINT
9. Viorel MOLDOVAN
10. Stephabe ZIANI
11. Nicolas SAVINAUD

SUBSTITUTES

8. Frederic DA ROCHA (19) 61
11. Pierre-Yves ANDRE (9) 76
16. Willy GRONDIN
17. Hassan AHAMADA
24. Yves DEROFF
25. Jean-Hugues BILAYI ATEBA (21) 79
31. Charles DEVINEAU

MATCH REPORT

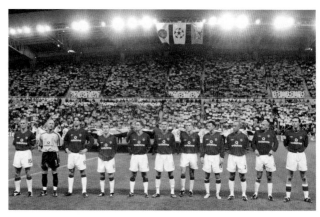

United line up to face the French champions in a potentially tricky tie

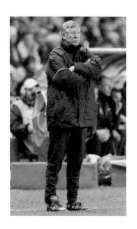

A penalty from Ruud van Nistelrooy in the fourth minute of added time saved the Red Devils from unexpected defeat after an avalanche of scoring chances had gone begging. Thanks largely to an inspired display by goalkeeper Landreau, the French champions looked set to claim the prized scalp of their English counterparts until Scholes' flick was handballed by Yepes, who was dismissed for a second bookable offence, and United's dead-eyed Dutchman netted emphatically from the

Sir Alex Ferguson looks on as Nantes put on an impressive first-half display in contrast to their disappointing domestic league form

1 MANCHESTER UNITED

90 VAN NISTELROOY (pen.)

1. Fabien BARTHEZ
2. Gary NEVILLE
27. Mikael SILVESTRE
4. Juan Sebastian VERON
12. Phil NEVILLE
6. Laurent BLANC
7. David BECKHAM
18. Paul SCHOLES
16. Roy KEANE
10. Ruud VAN NISTELROOY
11. Ryan GIGGS
SUBSTITUTES
3. Denis IRWIN
8. Nicky BUTT
13. Roy CARROLL
20. Ole Gunnar SOLSKJAER (4) 64
21. Diego FORLAN (12) 78
25. Quinton FORTUNE
30. John O'SHEA

spot. In fairness, Nantes had belied their recent disappointing domestic form with a potently enterprising first-half display and their early lead did not flatter them. True the goal involved an element of luck, the ball taking three deflections before Moldovan slipped it cleverly past Barthez from five yards. The former Coventry marksman had supplied the initial shot, which struck Blanc and fell to Quint, then his cross slid off both Beckham and Vahirua on its way to the scorer.

Thereafter the French continued to buzz and a horribly loose pass by Veron presaged a sinuous dribble and fierce shot by Vahirua, which brought a sterling save from Barthez. The Reds, though, were finding their range and van Nistelrooy threatened ceaselessly, going excruciatingly close to equalising when he swivelled and shot from 25 yards, only to see the ball rebound to safety from an upright. Next a Beckham volley brushed his toes at the far post, then he was through on Landreau, whose knee deflected the ball inches wide of goal. Vahirua might have doubled Nantes' advantage but his low shot was just off target; still United's dominance continued to build and Keane volleyed over from close range after being fed by Veron.

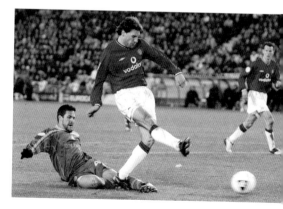

Ruud van Nistelrooy sidefoots the ball goalwards – only to see it rebound from the upright

MANCHESTER UNITED 1

VAN NISTELROOY 50

1. Fabien BARTHEZ
2. Gary NEVILLE
3. Denis IRWIN
4. Juan Sebastian VERON
27. Mikael SILVESTRE
6. Laurent BLANC
7. David BECKHAM
8. Nicky BUTT
20. Ole Gunnar SOLSKJAER
10. Ruud VAN NISTELROOY
16. Roy KEANE

SUBSTITUTES

5. Ronny JOHNSEN (3) 86
13. Roy CARROLL
18. Paul SCHOLES
21. Diego FORLAN
30. John O'SHEA

MATCH REPORT

A day which began with homage to Old Trafford's most revered goal king ended with gratitude to his modern equivalent. Prior to kick-off a statue of Denis Law was unveiled at the Stretford End, then Ruud van Nistelrooy's 29th strike of the season proved just enough to secure three crucial points towards the pursuit of yet another championship.

In testing conditions – a wickedly swirling wind and spongy, newly-laid turf – the Red Devils dominated territorially, but their shooting was so uncharacteristically wayward that returning hero Peter Schmeichel had remarkably few saves to make.

Keane, who went on to earn his customary man-of-the-match accolade, set the tone with an off-target drive after only 30 seconds, but it was something of a shock when the normally reliable van Nistelrooy squandered an inviting opportunity five minutes later. Veron created the opening with a sublimely flighted chip which was nodded down by Keane, only for the Dutchman to pull wide from 14 yards.

Villa were pinned back – though Angel managed one 30-yarder, straight at Barthez – and soon Veron fired wide twice, Schmeichel smothered at the feet of both Solskjaer and Beckham, and in

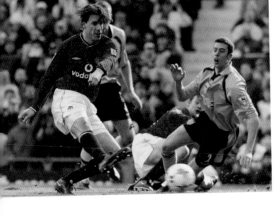

Ruud van Nistelrooy sidefoots home the only goal of the game early in the second half

0 ASTON VILLA

1. Peter SCHMEICHEL
2. Mark DELANEY
15. Gareth BARRY
4. Olof MELLBERG
31. Jlloyd SAMUEL
6. George BOATENG
22. Darius VASSELL
8. Juan Pablo ANGEL
20. Moustapha HADJI
18. Steve STONE
11. Steve STAUNTON

SUBSTITUTES

9. Dion DUBLIN (31) 79
12. Peter ENCKELMAN
19. Bosko BALABAN
21. Thomas HITZLSPERGER (20) 64
30. Hassan KACHLOUL

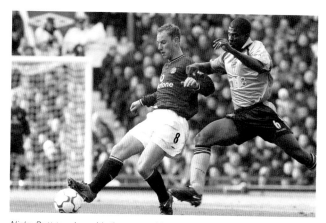

Nicky Butt tangles with the competitive George Boateng in an effort to control the midfield

yet another attack the Norwegian's shot was deflected for a corner by Mellberg. But the breakthrough was delayed until early in the second half when Boateng was robbed by Keane on the edge of the Villa box and the ball broke to van Nistelrooy, who swivelled to sidefoot into an empty net from 14 yards.

Almost immediately Beckham surged through the centre but shot narrowly high from 30 yards, then Schmeichel fielded a stinging Veron drive and van Nistelrooy scraped a post. Villa attempted a late rally, but Keane made a magnificent saving tackle on Angel and a Vassell dribble came to nothing, leaving United to keep possession imperiously as time ebbed away.

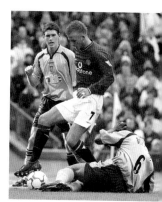

David Beckham dances his way through the Villa midfield

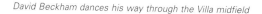

MANCHESTER UNITED 5

1. Fabien BARTHEZ
2. Gary NEVILLE
3. Denis IRWIN
4. Juan Sebastian VERON
27. Mikael SILVESTRE
6. Laurent BLANC
7. David BECKHAM
16. Roy KEANE
20. Ole Gunnar SOLSKJAER
10. Ruud VAN NISTELROOY
11. Ryan GIGGS

SUBSTITUTES

5. Ronny JOHNSEN (6) 69
8. Nicky BUTT (16) 75
12. Phil NEVILLE
13. Roy CARROLL
18. Paul SCHOLES
19. Dwight YORKE
21. Diego FORLAN (10) 69

BECKHAM 18
SOLSKJAER 31, 78
SILVESTRE 38
VAN NISTELROOY (pen.) 64

MATCH REPORT

The French champions were flattened comprehensively by the Red Devils' latest display of attacking football, though the margin of victory was a trifle less emphatic than the scoreline suggests. Going forward, United touched sublime heights, with Beckham at his most convincing and Solskjaer contributing a neat brace on his 29th birthday, but before claiming the points Sir Alex Ferguson's men suffered several defensive tremors. Indeed it was Nantes who dominated the first 15 minutes, retaining possession beautifully and creating several scoring chances. They almost took the lead when Cetto headed against the bar following a corner, then did so when the Reds failed to pick up Andre from a throw-in and his cross was converted clinically by Da Rocha from six yards.

Within a minute, though, United were level when Beckham curled a perfect free-kick over the wall from 28 yards, and the whole tenor of the contest changed. Now the hosts were on top and they made it pay when Irwin cut inside and passed to van Nistelrooy, who had roamed to the right flank; the Dutchman dispatched an inviting delivery to the far post, Giggs headed back across goal and there was Solskjaer to nod home from close range.

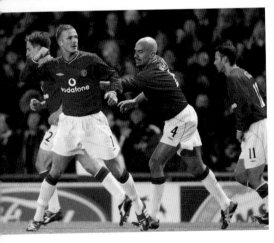

David Beckham celebrates his 18th-minute free-kick which effectively turned the game for United

1 NANTES ATLANTIQUE

17 DA ROCHA

1. Mickaël LANDREAU

2. Nestor FABBRI

25. Jean-Hugues BILAYI ATEBA

35. Mauro CETTO

22. Sylvain ARMAND

13. Mathieu BERSON

24. Yves DEROFF

8. Frederic DA ROCHA

20. Eric DJEMBA-DJEMBA

29. Stephane ZIANI

11. Pierre-Yves ANDRE

SUBSTITUTES

9. Viorel MOLDOVAN

15. Nicolas SAVINAUD (20) 57

16. Willy GRONDIN

17. Hassan AHAMADA

19. Marama VAHIRUA (25) 63

21. Olivier QUINT (29) 78

31. Charles DEVINEAU

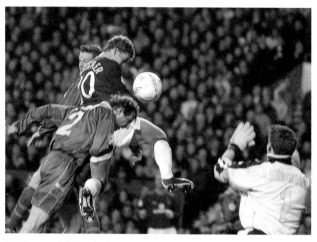

Ole Gunnar Solskjaer's downward header rounded off a splendid night for United against the French champions

Soon the rampant Reds struck again when Beckham's free-kick from the right was met by a booming header from Silvestre, though Da Rocha might have reduced the arrears shortly afterwards when he wriggled past two defenders before shooting against an upright from 20 yards. Nantes continued to counter-attack enterprisingly in the second period, but after Giggs shot against Landreau's post following a thrilling run there were two more United strikes to savour.

First van Nistelrooy netted powerfully from the spot after he was fouled by Fabbri, then Solskjaer met Beckham's arcing free-kick from the left with a glancing header to make it five.

FEBRUARY IN REVIEW

SATURDAY 2	v SUNDERLAND	A	4-1
SUNDAY 10	v CHARLTON ATHLETIC	A	2-0
WEDNESDAY 20	v NANTES ATLANTIQUE	A	1-1
SATURDAY 23	v ASTON VILLA	H	1-0
TUESDAY 26	v NANTES ATLANTIQUE	H	5-1

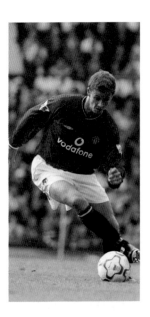

PLAYER IN THE FRAME

Ole Gunnar Solskjaer

A fabulous match-winning brace at Charlton and two more strikes at home to Nantes underlined Ole's inestimable value to the team. Not that there was much doubt about that, following his prolific midwinter exploits; it was just that the popular Norwegian appeared to grow ever more sharp as the season progressed. In addition to his goal-poaching, he contributed immensely by his willingness to forage tirelessly for possession. An absolute gem.

FA BARCLAYCARD PREMIERSHIP

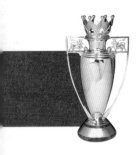

	P	W	D	L	F	A	Pts
MANCHESTER UNITED	28	18	3	7	67	35	57
Arsenal	27	15	9	3	55	31	54
Liverpool	28	15	8	5	45	25	53
Newcastle United	26	16	4	6	51	33	52
Chelsea	26	11	11	4	46	26	44
Leeds United	26	11	10	5	37	29	43
Aston Villa	27	9	11	7	32	30	38
Tottenham Hotspur	26	10	5	11	37	35	35
Fulham	27	8	11	8	27	29	35
West Ham United	27	9	7	11	30	42	34
Charlton Athletic	26	8	9	9	30	32	33
Middlesbrough	27	8	7	12	26	35	31
Sunderland	26	8	7	11	21	30	31
Southampton	27	9	4	14	31	41	31
Ipswich Town	26	8	6	12	34	40	30
Everton	27	7	8	12	27	34	29
Bolton Wanderers	27	6	11	10	30	42	29
Blackburn Rovers	26	6	7	13	32	36	25
Derby County	27	7	4	16	21	43	25
Leicester City	27	3	8	16	18	49	17

**UP TO AND INCLUDING
SATURDAY 23 FEBRUARY 2002**

MARCH

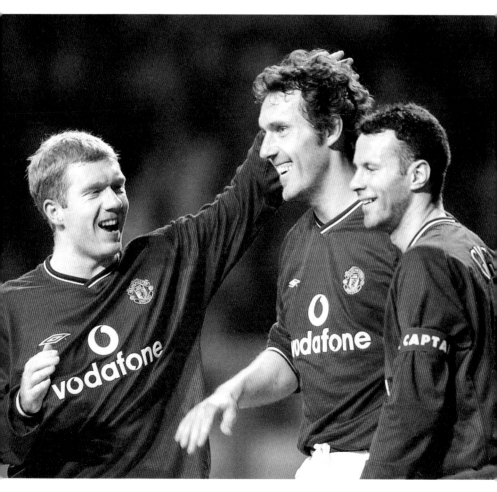

DERBY COUNTY 2

CHRISTIE 8, 78

24. Andy OAKES
22. Warren BARTON
16. Luciano ZAVAGNO
23. Paul BOERTIEN
15. Danny HIGGINBOTHAM
6. Chris RIGGOTT
7. Robert LEE
37. Pierre DUCROCQ
12. Malcolm CHRISTIE
10. Giorgi KINKLADZE
11. Fabrizio RAVANELLI

SUBSTITUTES

14. Lee MORRIS (37) 63
19. Steve ELLIOTT (10) 83
25. Branko STRUPAR (11) 75
27. Patrick FOLETTI
28. Simo VALAKARI

MATCH REPORT

Rarely can any team have dominated a game more comprehensively and yet failed to win than did Manchester United against relegation-threatened Derby. The Red Devils rapped the woodwork twice, had two vociferous penalty appeals denied and missed a hatful of chances, and yet this enthralling encounter might have ended on an even more disappointing note for Sir Alex Ferguson's men, who were indebted to the referee's controversial decision to disallow a late strike by Christie.

The game was awash with incident from the outset, with van Nistelrooy being flattened by Oakes in the act of heading narrowly wide in the second minute. Play was waved on, though, and the hosts enjoyed a brief period of command, during which Silvestre cleared off the line after Christie had shot from a narrow angle.

Derby went ahead when the ball bounced free for Christie to fire home from eight yards, and they might have doubled their lead eight minutes later when Kinkladze shaved a post, but that was the signal for the visitors to assume almost total superiority. Before the equaliser eventually materialised they went close to scoring seven times in 20 minutes, through van Nistelrooy (three

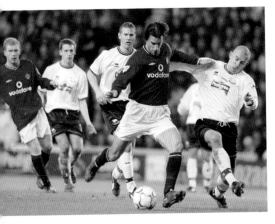

Ruud van Nistelrooy fails to take one of many scoring chances United made during the first half

2 MANCHESTER UNITED

41 SCHOLES
60 VERON

1. Fabien BARTHEZ
2. Gary NEVILLE
3. Denis IRWIN
4. Juan Sebastian VERON
5. Ronny JOHNSEN
27. Mikael SILVESTRE
7. David BECKHAM
18. Paul SCHOLES
20. Ole Gunnar SOLSKJAER
10. Ruud VAN NISTELROOY
11. Ryan GIGGS
SUBSTITUTES
8. Nicky BUTT
12. Phil NEVILLE
13. Roy CARROLL
21. Diego FORLAN (11) 80
30. John O'SHEA (3) 84

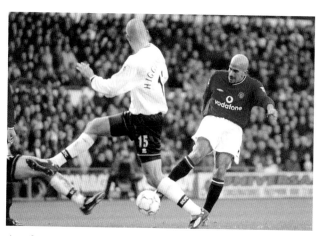

Juan Sebastian Veron shoots from the edge of the box to give United a 2-1 lead on the hour mark

times), Beckham, Solskjaer (who shot against an upright), Giggs and Scholes. That intense pressure finally told when Giggs reached the byline and pulled the ball back for Scholes to crash in from six yards.

After the break the one-sided story continued with Beckham (twice) and van Nistelrooy, whose shot on the turn was saved by Oakes, almost breaking through. United took a richly deserved lead through Veron's scudding 20-yarder and the outcome seemed a formality. But then Christie turned in Zavagno's cross at the near post and the impressively mobile marksman so nearly won the game at the death, but was judged to have robbed Barthez unfairly before poking into an empty net.

MANCHESTER UNITED 4

BECKHAM 15, 64
VAN NISTELROOY 43 (pen.), 76

1. Fabien BARTHEZ
2. Gary NEVILLE
27. Mikael SILVESTRE
4. Juan Sebastian VERON
5. Ronny JOHNSEN
6. Laurent BLANC
7. David BECKHAM
18. Paul SCHOLES
21. Diego FORLAN
10. Ruud VAN NISTELROOY
16. Roy KEANE

SUBSTITUTES

8. Nicky BUTT (18) 71
11. Ryan GIGGS
12. Phil NEVILLE (2) 69
13. Roy CARROLL
25. Quinton FORTUNE (4) 71

MATCH REPORT

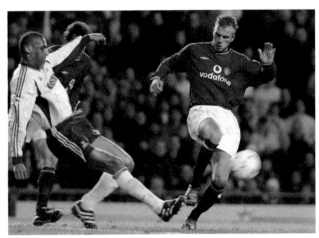

David Beckham is unable to add to his two-goal tally as Spurs defender Dean Richards takes the ball off his toes

David Beckham and Ruud van Nistelrooy each grabbed a brace as the imperious Reds swept aside ten-man Tottenham to return to the Premiership peak. In the end, United strolled to victory, but their progress was eased by the dismissal of Taricco shortly before the interval for holding back Scholes. Subsequent TV evidence revealed that the offence was committed outside the box, but van Nistelrooy netted from the spot to give his side a daunting 2-0 advantage from which the Londoners never looked likely to recover.

0 TOTTENHAM HOTSPUR

1. Neil SULLIVAN
18. Ben THATCHER
3. Mauricio TARICCO
23. Christian ZIEGE
36. Dean RICHARDS
26. Ledley KING
29. Simon DAVIES
8. Tim SHERWOOD
14. Gustavo POYET
10. Teddy SHERINGHAM
11. Sergei REBROV

SUBSTITUTES

6. Chris PERRY (14) 66
9. Les FERDINAND (11) h-t
13. Kasey KELLER
28. Matthew ETHERINGTON (23) 86
30. Anthony GARDNER

Spurs had begun the game purposefully and Barthez was required to make an athletic early save from a Poyet 20-yarder, but then the hosts took the lead with a beautifully worked goal. Beckham found van Nistelrooy on the right, outpaced Thatcher for the return ball and dispatched a low left-footer just inside the far post from 12 yards. Seconds later Scholes sent in van Nistelrooy, who rounded Sullivan and netted, only to be ruled offside.

Then came the penalty and the game became almost totally one-sided. True, Ferdinand might have done better than volley skywards at the start of the second period, but after that the Reds created chance after chance, beginning with a Blanc long-distance drive which brought a plunging parry from Sullivan.

A sub-plot to the contest was Forlan's bid to mark his first start with a goal but, despite a lively display, he failed to register. However, he compensated by outsprinting Richards on the left and crossing to his Dutch strike partner, who touched the ball on for Beckham to score from 15 yards.

All that remained was for van Nistelrooy to pounce when Sullivan palmed out a Keane centre; his 32nd goal of the season coming after his shimmy had mesmerised three defenders.

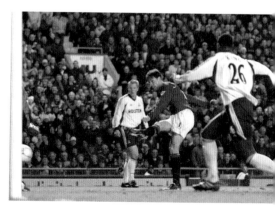

A static Spurs defence can only stand and admire as Ruud van Nistelrooy makes it 4-0

MANCHESTER UNITED   0

1. Fabien BARTHEZ
2. Gary NEVILLE
27. Mikael SILVESTRE
4. Juan Sebastian VERON
5. Ronny JOHNSEN
6. Laurent BLANC
7. David BECKHAM
16. Roy KEANE
20. Ole Gunnar SOLSKJAER
10. Ruud VAN NISTELROOY
11. Ryan GIGGS

SUBSTITUTES

3. Denis IRWIN
8. Nicky BUTT
12. Phil NEVILLE
13. Roy CARROLL
18. Paul SCHOLES
21. Diego FORLAN (20) 78
25. Quinton FORTUNE

MATCH REPORT

Two multi-talented teams served up numbingly drab fare for long stretches of a largely arid contest, but in the end the Red Devils did what was required of them to advance to the quarter-finals of the Champions League for a record sixth successive season. In all fairness, after three years without a goalless draw at Old Trafford the home fans fans could hardly complain about one goalless encounter, and come the final whistle they were rejoicing at the prospect of another tilt at European glory.

The first half was particularly dull, with Bayern withdrawing 11 men behind the ball at the merest hint of danger. The only man who hinted at breaching that formidable barrier was Giggs,

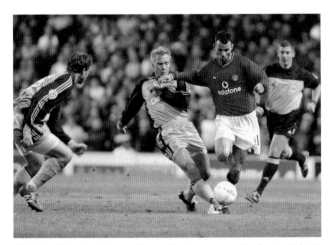

Only Ryan Giggs looked remotely capable of opening up the Bayern defence

0 BAYERN MUNICH

1. Oliver KAHN
25. Thomas LINKE
3. Bixente LIZARAZU
4. Samuel KUFFOUR
12. Robert KOVAC
16. Jens JEREMIES
23. Owen HARGREAVES
24. Roque SANTA CRUZ
14. Claudio PIZARRO
13. PAULO SERGIO
11. Stefan EFFENBERG

SUBSTITUTES

2. Willy SAGNOL
9. Giovane ELBER (13) 83
10. Ciriaco SFORZA
17. Thorsten FINK (16) 73
18. Michael TARNAT
21. Alexander ZICKLER (24) 77
22. Bernd DREHER

who shot wide after one jinking run, and sent in van Nistelrooy and Solskjaer, only for both marksmen to be ruled offside.

The second period opened more promisingly, with Giggs catching the eye once more when he wrong-footed Kuffour and brought a full-length parry from Kahn with a low drive from the edge of the box. Next the Welshman delivered a cross which was nodded wide by van Nistelrooy, encouraging hopes of a concerted United assault, but what materialised was a brief period of frenetic pressure from the Germans. In quick succession Barthez saved an eight-yard header from Pizarro, a Jeremies 25-yarder and a mishit volley by Effenberg. The Reds retaliated when Beckham's floater found van Nistelrooy and the Dutchman's 18-yard scorcher was repelled by Kahn, the rebound spinning to safety.

That might have been the prelude to a nerve-tingling finale, but far from it. Instead both teams played it safe with lengthy passing interludes in non-threatening areas, and the game fizzled out as tamely as it had begun. It was a fair bet that any meeting between the pair in later stages of the competition would be rather more lively.

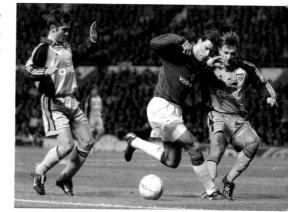

Even the quick-footed Ruud van Nistelrooy was unable to find a way through

WEST HAM UNITED 3

1. David JAMES
2. Tomas REPKA
3. Nigel WINTERBURN
30. Sebastien SCHEMMEL
5. Vladimir LABANT
26. Joe COLE
7. Christian DAILLY
21. Michael CARRICK
14. Frederic KANOUTE
10. Paolo DI CANIO
11. Steve LOMAS

SUBSTITUTES

16. John MONCUR
17. Shaka HISLOP
19. Ian PEARCE
25. Jermain DEFOE (3) 74
33. Richard GARCIA

LOMAS 8
KANOUTE 20
DEFOE 78

MATCH REPORT

Here was a sporting contest of rare splendour. After being dislodged from the Premiership pinnacle for some three hours by Liverpool, the Red Devils regained their perch with a captivating display of attacking football against enterprising opponents who also contributed mightily to the entertainment feast. The drama began early and never flagged, with United tearing forward insistently, but it was West Ham who struck first when Labant's cross from the left was met by Lomas' ferocious 14-yard header, which appeared to catch Barthez unawares.

Thus encouraged, the Hammers returned to the offensive and Labant went close, but then Upton Park was illuminated by a sequence of sheer, unadulterated beauty. Cole's wayward pass was controlled by Scholes, who delivered an instant raking dispatch into the path of Beckham on the right. Without breaking stride the England captain chipped over the stranded James from the corner of the box to equalise in world-class style. Unbowed, the Hammers hit back almost at once as Schemmel swept down the right and centred for Kanoute to sidefoot home from 18 yards. But their latest lead was short-lived as Beckham's free-kick was met by Butt's horizontal close-range volley. End-to-end action filled the remainder of a pulsating first half, but the Reds took command in

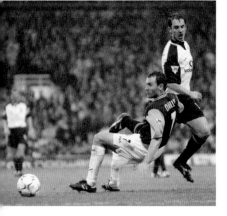

Gary Neville races past Christian Dailly on one of his many forays into the West Ham half

5   MANCHESTER UNITED

17, 89 (pen.) BECKHAM
22 BUTT
55 SCHOLES
64 SOLSKJAER

1. Fabien BARTHEZ
2. Gary NEVILLE
27. Mikael SILVESTRE
16. Roy KEANE
5. Ronny JOHNSEN
6. Laurent BLANC
7. David BECKHAM
8. Nicky BUTT
20. Ole Gunnar SOLSKJAER
10. Ruud VAN NISTELROOY
18. Paul SCHOLES
SUBSTITUTES
3. Denis IRWIN
12. Phil NEVILLE
13. Roy CARROLL
21. Diego FORLAN (20) 84
25. Quinton FORTUNE (10) 87

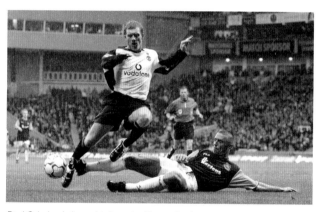

Paul Scholes is brought down by Tomas Repka...

the second and nosed ahead when Scholes turned Solskjaer's pull-back into an empty net. The visitors continued to dominate and appeared to have entered the comfort zone when the Norwegian clipped in from an acute angle, and then continued to fashion further scoring chances.

But the hosts were not done and Defoe stabbed in a cross from Kanoute, then had a penalty claim turned down. However, the referee could hardly miss Repka's felling of Scholes and Beckham netted explosively from the spot to ensure a classic victory.

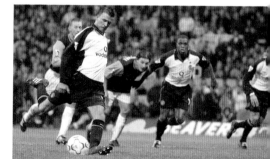

... and David Beckham buries the resultant penalty to ensure United take the spoils

BOAVISTA   0

1. RICARDO
23. Nuno Miguel FRECHAUT
25. Armando PETIT
4. PAULO TURRA
5. PEDRO EMANUEL
19. MARIO LOJA
7. JORGE SILVA
8. DUDA
9. SERGINHO
37. SANCHEZ
11. SILVA

SUBSTITUTES

3. Fernando AVALOS
10. MARCIO SANTOS (30) 59
16. MARTELINHO (7) 34
18. PEDRO SANTOS
20. JORGE COUTO
24. KHADIM Faye
30. Alexandre GOULART (11) 21

MATCH REPORT

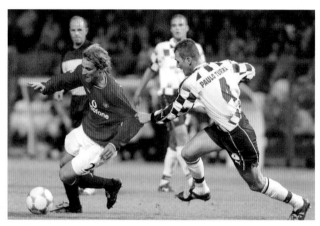

Diego Forlan was at the centre of most of United's play, but was unable to register his first goal for the club despite several chances

The Red Devils thumped the Portuguese champions comprehensively on their own turf to ensure top spot in their qualifying group. Hard-working Boavista did not just lie down and die, being desperate to prove their elimination from the competition was no reflection on their quality, but they hardly helped their case by gifting a soft early goal to United when Ricardo failed to claim a Beckham corner and the unattended Blanc sidefooted home from six yards.

Thus boosted, the visitors almost doubled their lead when Forlan ignored the risk of possible decapitation by a defender's

3 MANCHESTER UNITED

14 BLANC
29 SOLSKJAER
51 (pen.) BECKHAM

1. Fabien BARTHEZ
2. Gary NEVILLE
27. Mikael SILVESTRE
18. Paul SCHOLES
5. Ronny JOHNSEN
6. Laurent BLANC
7. David BECKHAM
8. Nicky BUTT
20. Ole Gunnar SOLSKJAER
21. Diego FORLAN
11. Ryan GIGGS

SUBSTITUTES

3. Denis IRWIN
12. Phil NEVILLE (5) 73
13. Roy CARROLL
25. Quinton FORTUNE
28. Michael STEWART (18) 59
30. John O'SHEA (6) 73
32. Bojan DJORDJIC

flailing boot to launch himself at a Giggs cross, only for Ricardo to parry his close-range header. That moment was to sum up a frustrating night for the unlucky Uruguayan, who performed splendidly but just could not notch his first goal for the club.

Boavista responded with gusto and Sanchez swerved past Butt before hitting a 25-yard curler which brought a fine save from Barthez. However, the most fluent football continued to flow from the Reds and they might have scored again when a Forlan thunderbolt was pushed out by Ricardo into the path of Beckham, only for the England skipper to blaze over.

Next a Forlan cross was nodded over by Solskjaer, but then the Norwegian supplied the inevitable second goal when he seized on a rebound to net from six yards following a slick interchange between Beckham and Giggs. United's third arrived early in the second half when Butt burst through the centre and chipped to Scholes, who was tripped by Martelinho. Beckham netted from the spot and might have been asked to do so again, but the blatant felling of Gary Neville went unpunished.

Thereafter Ricardo repelled a Stewart screamer, Barthez acrobatically foiled Serginho and the Reds were left to contemplate the quarter-finals.

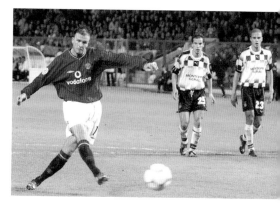

David Beckham scores from the spot much to the disappointment of the Boavista defence

MANCHESTER UNITED 0

- 1. Fabien BARTHEZ
- 2. Gary NEVILLE
- 27. Mikael SILVESTRE
- 4. Juan Sebastian VERON
- 5. Ronny JOHNSEN
- 6. Laurent BLANC
- 7. David BECKHAM
- 8. Nicky BUTT
- 21. Diego FORLAN
- 10. Ruud VAN NISTELROOY
- 11. Ryan GIGGS

SUBSTITUTES

- 12. Phil NEVILLE
- 13. Roy CARROLL
- 18. Paul SCHOLES (4) 59
- 25. Quinton FORTUNE (21) 83
- 30. John O'SHEA

MATCH REPORT

On an afternoon of unremitting frustration, the Red Devils lost crucial ground in the Championship race. The only goal of a frantic contest was gifted to feisty, well-organised Middlesbrough by Veron, who received his biggest cheer when he was replaced by the popular Scholes midway through the second half. United had their chances and they enjoyed plenty of possession, but it was telling that the hosts' most impressive figure, by some distance, was the immaculate Blanc.

The decisive breakthrough came when the £28 million Argentinian dithered in possession and was robbed by Carbone. The Italian, who excelled throughout, strode forward and squared a simple ball for Boksic to stroke neatly past the exposed Barthez from eight yards. United retaliated briskly with Beckham and Giggs combining to find Forlan on the right, his cross was controlled sweetly by van Nistelrooy, but a shot on the turn flashed inches wide. Next Beckham cut infield and found Giggs unmarked on the left, but the Welshman also fired wide.

Middlesbrough might have extended their lead when Boksic eluded his markers to meet Carbone's chip, only to miscue from the corner of the six-yard box, but most of the pressure came from United and the half ended with a flying Forlan volley which cleared the angle.

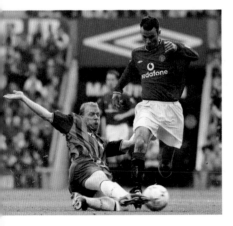

Ryan Giggs was at the heart of most of United's attacks, but the Welshman was unable to make the breakthrough

1 MIDDLESBROUGH

9 BOKSIC

1. Mark SCHWARZER	
27. Robbie STOCKDALE	
37. Franck QUEUDRUE	
12. Jonathan GREENING	
17. Ugo EHIOGU	
6. Gareth SOUTHGATE	
7. Robbie MUSTOE	
26. Noel WHELAN	
9. Paul INCE	
10. Benito CARBONE	
11. Alen BOKSIC	

SUBSTITUTES

8. Szilard NEMETH
25. Mark CROSSLEY
20. Dean WINDASS (11) 79
29. Jason GAVIN
31. Luke WILKSHIRE (12) 21

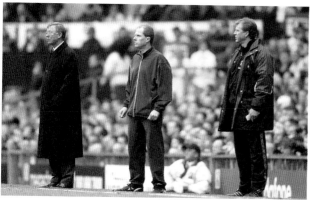

Sir Alex Ferguson and Steve McClaren watch the action unfold

The Reds pushed forward throughout the second period, fashioning a series of openings but the customary conviction and cutting edge were lacking. In quick succession van Nistelrooy headed over from crosses by Silvestre and Beckham, then Neville's nod from Giggs' dispatch also went adrift. Scholes drove wide from 20 yards before the England midfielder opened Boro with a beautiful floater which sent in van Nistelrooy, only for Schwarzer to block brilliantly from close range. That summed up United's disappointing day.

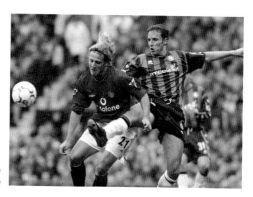

Diego Forlan feels the power of Gareth Southgate's tackling

LEEDS UNITED 3

1. Nigel MARTYN
18. Danny MILLS
3. Ian HARTE
23. David BATTY
21. Dominic MATTEO
6. Jonathan WOODGATE
17. Alan SMITH
27. Robbie FOWLER
9. Mark VIDUKA
10. Harry KEWELL
20. Seth JOHNSON

SUBSTITUTES

2. Gary KELLY
7. Robbie KEANE (20) 65
11. Lee BOWYER (10) 12
13. Paul ROBINSON
19. Eirik BAKKE (23) 60

VIDUKA 20
HARTE 62
BOWYER 80

MATCH REPORT

They did it the hard way in the end, but the swashbuckling Reds kept alive their Championship hopes in an enthralling seven-goal cliffhanger. Leading 4-1 shortly after the interval, they appeared to be in the comfort zone, but Leeds surged back courageously and the visitors were clinging on at the final whistle.

After the game had begun at a predictably furious tempo, the Reds struck the first blow when a deliciously subtle Scholes nudge guided the ball to Silvestre on the left; he beat Mills and crossed for the England midfielder to thump past Martyn from 12 yards. Leeds responded with a wave of pressure, with Harte and Fowler volleying wide before Bowyer freed Viduka to clip a neat equaliser. The Reds might have regained their lead almost immediately but Silvestre headed narrowly wide from a Beckham corner, then Scholes' exquisite instant pass sent Keane into the Leeds box, only for the skipper to stumble.

However, they seized the initiative in compelling manner with two Solskjaer strikes inside two minutes. First Giggs backheeled to Scholes, whose 25-yard dipper was pushed out by Martyn to the Norwegian, who pounced to net from the left corner of the six-yard area. Next Silvestre centred from the byline and the ball ran free to Solskjaer, whose low drive went in via a deflection.

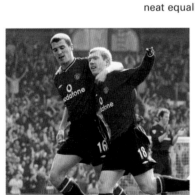

Skipper Roy Keane congratulates Paul Scholes after his ninth-minute goal had given United the lead

4 MANCHESTER UNITED

9 SCHOLES
37, 39 SOLSKJAER
54 GIGGS

1. Fabien BARTHEZ	
2. Gary NEVILLE	
27. Mikael SILVESTRE	
16. Roy KEANE	
5. Ronny JOHNSEN	
6. Laurent BLANC	
7. David BECKHAM	
8. Nicky BUTT	
20. Ole Gunnar SOLSKJAER	
18. Paul SCHOLES	
11. Ryan GIGGS	
SUBSTITUTES	
3. Denis IRWIN	
10. Ruud VAN NISTELROOY	
12. Phil NEVILLE (20) 86	
13. Roy CARROLL	
21. Diego FORLAN (11) 75	

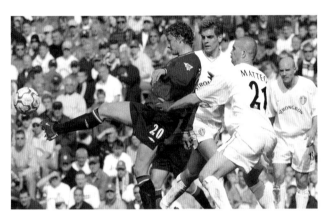

Ole Gunnar Solskjaer nets a rebound to restore United's lead

The second half began with Sir Alex Ferguson's men in full command, and it wasn't long before the fourth goal arrived. Blanc broke up a Leeds raid and found Beckham, who sprinted half the length of the field before setting up Giggs to stab home from ten yards.

The Reds attacked again and though Johnsen's header rebounded from the Leeds bar, the result seemed a formality. But now the hosts rallied gamely, and a 30-yard Harte free-kick and Bowyer's nod from Fowler's miscue set up a photo-finish.

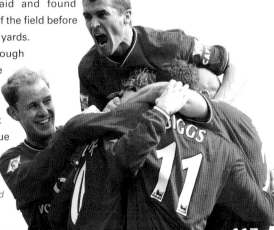

Roy Keane leads the celebrations as United take a two-goal lead

MARCH IN REVIEW

SUNDAY 3	v DERBY COUNTY	A	2-2
WEDNESDAY 6	v TOTTENHAM HOTSPUR	A	4-0
WEDNESDAY 13	v BAYERN MUNICH	H	0-0
SATURDAY 16	v WEST HAM UNITED	A	5-3
TUESDAY 19	v BOAVISTA	A	3-0
SATURDAY 23	v MIDDLESBROUGH	H	0-1
SATURDAY 30	v LEEDS UNITED	A	4-3

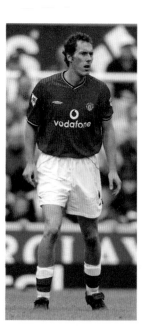

PLAYER IN THE FRAME

Laurent Blanc

Though Sir Alex Ferguson had spoken highly of the veteran Frenchman, he had come in for some criticism. By the spring, though, Laurent's class and composure finally began to tell, and especially against Spurs and Bayern Munich at Old Trafford when he was utterly imperious. For good measure he added the opening goal against Boavista, and suddenly there was speculation about a new contract.

FA BARCLAYCARD PREMIERSHIP

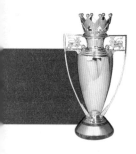

UP TO AND INCLUDING
SATURDAY 30 MARCH 2002

	P	W	D	L	F	A	Pts
Liverpool	33	20	8	5	55	26	68
MANCHESTER UNITED	33	21	4	8	82	44	67
Arsenal	31	19	9	3	63	32	66
Newcastle United	31	18	5	8	60	42	59
Chelsea	32	15	11	6	60	32	56
Leeds United	32	14	12	6	47	34	54
Aston Villa	32	10	12	10	37	39	42
Tottenham Hotspur	32	12	6	14	42	46	42
Charlton Athletic	32	10	11	11	35	38	41
West Ham United	31	11	7	13	38	50	40
Middlesbrough	32	10	9	13	31	39	39
Southampton	32	10	8	14	39	47	38
Fulham	32	8	12	12	31	39	36
Everton	32	9	9	14	35	45	36
Bolton Wanderers	32	8	12	12	37	50	36
Sunderland	32	9	8	15	24	41	35
Blackburn Rovers	31	8	8	15	40	43	32
Ipswich Town	32	8	8	16	39	52	32
Derby County	32	8	5	19	30	53	29
Leicester City	32	4	10	18	23	56	22

APRIL

TUESDAY 2	**v DEPORTIVO LA CORUÑA A**
SATURDAY 6	**v LEICESTER CITY A**
WEDNESDAY 10	**v DEPORTIVO LA CORUÑA H**
SATURDAY 20	**v CHELSEA A**
WEDNESDAY 24	**v BAYER 04 LEVERKUSEN H**
SATURDAY 27	**v IPSWICH TOWN A**
TUESDAY 30	**v BAYER 04 LEVERKUSEN A**

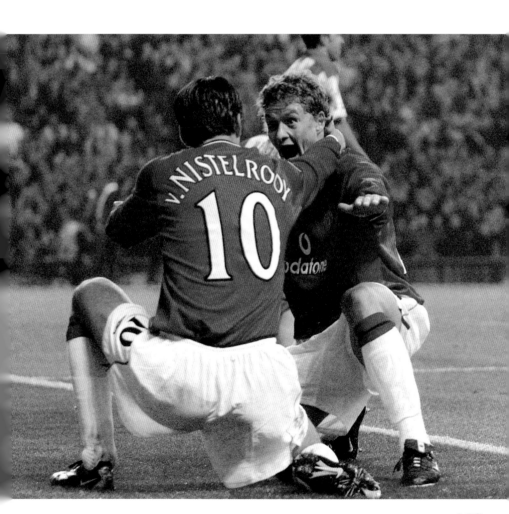

DEPORTIVO LA CORUÑA   0

1. Francisco MOLINA
12. Lionel SCALONI
3. Enrique ROMERO
4. Nourredine NAYBET
5. CESAR Martin
6. MAURO SILVA
18. VICTOR Sanchez
21. Juan Carlos VALERON
9. Diego TRISTAN
10. FRAN Gonzalez
16. SERGIO

SUBSTITUTES

7. Roy MAKAAY (10) 60
8. DJALMINHA (21) 68
13. NUNO Simoes
15. Joan CAPDEVILA
17. Walter PANDIANI
23. Aldo Pedro DUSCHER (18) 87
24. HECTOR

MATCH REPORT

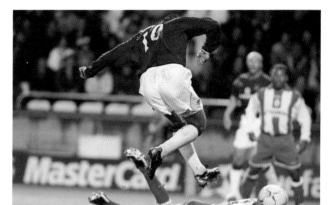

Ruud van Nistelrooy sidefoots the ball home to put United two up...

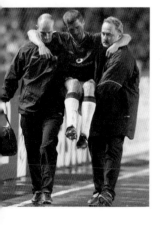

Manchester United comprehensively outplayed one of the Champions League favourites, giving arguably their most convincing European performance for many a season. However, the celebrations were soured by an ominous-looking injury to the inspirational Keane and a hefty late knock to Beckham, a double blow rendered all the more serious by a booking which would remove Scholes from the second leg.

With Giggs given a free role and Scholes starting on the left, United began fluently and took the lead in sensational fashion. There seemed little danger when Beckham accepted a pass from

A disconsolate Roy Keane is carried off moments before half time

2 MANCHESTER UNITED

15 BECKHAM
41 VAN NISTELROOY

1. Fabien BARTHEZ
2. Gary NEVILLE
27. Mikael SILVESTRE
16. Roy KEANE
5. Ronny JOHNSEN
6. Laurent BLANC
7. David BECKHAM
8. Nicky BUTT
18. Paul SCHOLES
10. Ruud VAN NISTELROOY
11. Ryan GIGGS
SUBSTITUTES
3. Denis IRWIN
12. Phil NEVILLE (7) 90
13. Roy CARROLL
20. Ole Gunnar SOLSKJAER (10) 76
21. Diego FORLAN
25. Quinton FORTUNE (16) 45
30. John O'SHEA

Keane some 35 yards out, but the England captain unleashed a looping chip of such unerring accuracy that Molina was beaten, though he was only marginally off his line. The Reds doubled their advantage when Johnsen found Silvestre on the left and the Frenchman's cross was sidefooted home by van Nistelrooy.

Keane was stretchered away before the interval but United's command did not relent in the second period, when apparent penalty-box misdemeanours on Silvestre and van Nistelrooy went unpunished, Giggs saw one effort cleared off the line by Cesar and another blocked by Molina, and Solskjaer was denied by the woodwork. With Deportivo reduced mainly to shooting from distance, the Reds' second Champions League victory on Spanish soil – the first was in the 1999 final – duly materialised.

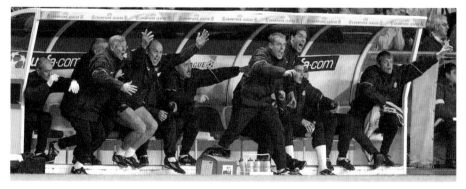

... and the Red's bench shows its delight

LEICESTER CITY   0

16. Ian WALKER

2. Gary ROWETT

3. Frank SINCLAIR

17. Stefan OAKES

18. Matt ELLIOTT

14. Callum DAVIDSON

29. Matthew PIPER

8. Robbie SAVAGE

22. Paul DICKOV

27. Brian DEANE

26. Lee MARSHALL

SUBSTITUTES

1. Tim FLOWERS

28. Matthew HEATH

32. Jon STEVENSON

33. Martin REEVES (17) 80

35. Jon ASHTON (14) 83

MATCH REPORT

One flash of supreme class by master marksman Ole Gunnar Solskjaer in an otherwise arid contest was enough to lift the Red Devils back to the Premiership peak – albeit only until teatime – and condemn gallant Leicester to relegation.

    With the swirling wind and bumpy pitch rendering their customary slick-passing game untenable, and with a bevy of star performers either injured or benched, United were nowhere near their best, and might have been trailing long before they snatched the game's solitary goal. That they weren't was due largely to a combination of splendid goalkeeping by Carroll and errant finishing from the Foxes, who created and spurned several clear scoring opportunities. The Irishman's first timely intervention came in the third minute when Piper's cross fell to Deane, who hammered the ball goalwards from close range, only for Carroll to smother courageously, and he was equally adept in repelling an awkward Dickov cross-shot midway through the first half.

    The Reds responded with a hopeful dink from Forlan and two long-range efforts from Scholes, none of which registered, before Dickov went perilously close with a four-yard volley shortly before the break.

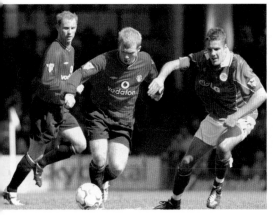

Paul Scholes tidies up in midfield

1 MANCHESTER UNITED

61 SOLSKJAER

12. Roy CARROLL
2. Gary NEVILLE
3. Denis IRWIN
12. Phil NEVILLE
27. Mikael SILVESTRE
6. Laurent BLANC
18. Paul SCHOLES
8. Nicky BUTT
20. Ole Gunnar SOLSKJAER
21. Diego FORLAN
25. Quinton FORTUNE
SUBSTITUTES
10. Ruud VAN NISTELROOY (25) 51
11. Ryan GIGGS (21) 63
17. Raimond VAN DER GOUW
24. Wesley BROWN (3) 78
30. John O'SHEA

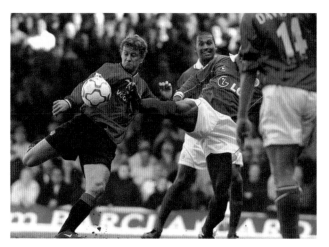

Despite a wall of Leicester City defenders, Ole Gunnar Solskjaer is able to control the ball on his chest before drilling it past Ian Walker

Early in the second half Leicester had a penalty appeal turned down, then Deane missed with a free header from 12 yards before the visitors, reinforced by the arrival of van Nistelrooy and Giggs, finally mounted a spell of pressure which culminated in the breakthrough. Phil Neville's long throw from the right was touched on to Solskjaer, who controlled the ball on his chest and swivelled to net with a scorching volley from 12 yards.

Thereafter the Reds looked a little more like themselves, with van Nistelrooy twice going close and Scholes bringing a flying save from Walker with a ferocious 20-yarder. In the end, though it had not been pretty, they had done enough.

MANCHESTER UNITED 3

1. Fabien BARTHEZ
2. Gary NEVILLE
27. Mikael SILVESTRE
4. Juan Sebastian VERON
5. Ronny JOHNSEN
6. Laurent BLANC
7. David BECKHAM
8. Nicky BUTT
25. Quinton FORTUNE
10. Ruud VAN NISTELROOY
11. Ryan GIGGS
SUBSTITUTES
3. Denis IRWIN
12. Phil NEVILLE (4) 74
13. Roy CARROLL
20. Ole Gunnar SOLSKJAER (7) 21
21. Diego FORLAN
24. Wesley BROWN (5) 37
28. Michael STEWART

SOLSKJAER 23, 56
GIGGS 69

MATCH REPORT

The Red Devils marched imperiously into the last four of the Champions League on a night when Veron offered an eloquent riposte to his critics, Solskjaer was his usual predatory self and Giggs, the new skipper in Keane's absence, contributed a goal of true majesty. Sadly, as in the first leg when the Irishman was crocked, injury to key players took the edge off the celebrations. This time the victims were Beckham, his foot broken by a wild tackle from Duscher, and Johnsen, who damaged a hamstring.

As for Deportivo, they performed with their customary fluency, but were well beaten by the time they were reduced to nine men through the second-half dismissals of Scaloni and Duscher, each for repeated bookable offences.

In an entertainingly open match, the Reds began purposefully and might have broken through after ten minutes when Fortune seized on a weak clearance but Molina parried athletically. Then, with the action flowing from end to end, Barthez saved superbly at Tristan's feet and van Nistelrooy was crowded out by Hector. Soon Beckham was stretchered away but United spirits were lifted when Veron speared a free-kick into the box and newly-arrived substitute Solskjaer volleyed home from six yards.

The Spaniards equalised when Romero's low cross from the left was diverted past Barthez by

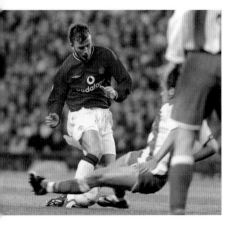

David Beckham is on the receiving end of a dangerous tackle from Deportivo's Aldo Pedro Duscher

2 DEPORTIVO LA CORUÑA

45 BLANC (o.g.)
90 DJALMINHA

1. Francisco MOLINA
12. Lionel SCALONI
3. Enrique ROMERO
4. Nourredine NAYBET
24. HECTOR
21. Juan Carlos VALERON
18. VICTOR Sanchez
8. DJALMINHA
9. Diego TRISTAN
10. FRAN Gonzalez
23. Aldo Pedro DUSCHER

SUBSTITUTES

7. Roy MAKAAY (18) 51
11. Jose Emilio AMAVISCA
13. NUNO Simoes
14. EMERSON
15. Joan CAPDEVILA (10) 63
17. Walter PANDIANI (9) 73
25. JOSE MANUEL

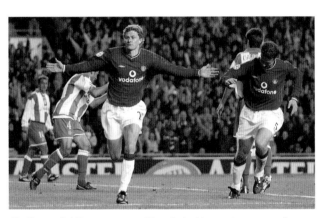

Ole Gunnar Solskjaer announces his arrival with a goal moments after coming on as a substitute for David Beckham

Blanc, but the Reds might have regained their lead when van Nistelrooy headed wide from a Giggs cross shortly before the break. Victory was virtually assured, though, when Veron found Solskjaer and the Norwegian deceived Molina with his narrow-angled shot.

Next the Argentinian freed Giggs, who hared down the right, cut inside past two defenders and netted with an unstoppable left-footer. Thereafter van Nistelrooy nodded against the bar and Djalminha scored with a deflected free-kick, but by then it didn't matter.

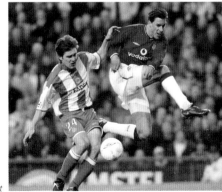

Ruud van Nistelrooy fails to connect with a right-foot shot

CHELSEA 0

23. Carlo CUDICINI

15. Mario MELCHIOT

13. William GALLAS

17. Emmanuel PETIT

26. John TERRY

6. Marcel DESAILLY

30. Jesper GRONKJAER

8. Frank LAMPARD

9. Jimmy Floyd HASSELBAINK

22. Eidur GUDJOHNSEN

25. Gianfranco ZOLA

SUBSTITUTES

1. Ed DE GOEY

10. Slavisa JOKANOVIC

11. Boudewijn ZENDEN (22) h-t

24. Samuelle DALLA BONA (17) 78

29. Robert HUTH

MATCH REPORT

The Red Devils exacted fitting revenge for their demoralising December drubbing at the hands of the Blues, neatly reversing the Old Trafford scoreline and preserving their title aspirations. In truth, Claudio Ranieri's men subsided limply and United were cruising towards victory from the moment Scholes opened the scoring with a 30-yard bombshell, fired after Giggs had wrong-footed the Chelsea rearguard with a disguised free-kick from the right.

The heart seemed to have deserted the FA Cup finalists and with Butt and Scholes commanding centre-field, it came as no surprise when the Reds struck again, Gary Neville and Giggs combining neatly before Solskjaer slipped an exquisite pass to

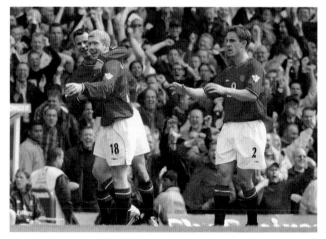

Paul Scholes accepts the congratulations after giving United the lead

3 MANCHESTER UNITED

15 SCHOLES
41 VAN NISTELROOY
86 SOLSKJAER

1. Fabien BARTHEZ
2. Gary NEVILLE
27. Mikael SILVESTRE
18. Paul SCHOLES
5. Wesley BROWN
6. Laurent BLANC
25. Quinton FORTUNE
8. Nicky BUTT
20. Ole Gunnar SOLSKJAER
10. Ruud VAN NISTELROOY
11. Ryan GIGGS
SUBSTITUTES
3. Denis IRWIN
12. Phil NEVILLE (25) 41
13. Roy CARROLL
21. Diego FORLAN (11) 87
30. John O'SHEA

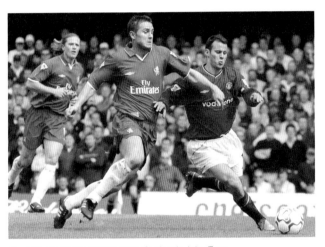

Ryan Giggs forces his way past Chelsea's John Terry

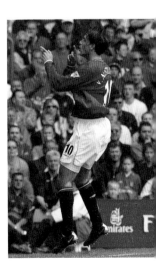

van Nistelrooy. This time the Dutchman made no mistake, dancing around Cudicini and netting from a narrow angle.

Five minutes after the break Lampard brought a comfortable stop from Barthez, and that was virtually the end of the hosts as an attacking force. United, meanwhile, assumed serene control and only the excellence of Cudicini prevented a third goal when he repelled a Giggs drive with his feet, then sprang from the ground to divert van Nistelrooy's follow-up. But even the agile Italian was helpless to prevent the Reds completing the rout when van Nistelrooy gulled Desailly on the left and switched inside to Giggs, who set up Solskjaer for a far-post finish.

Ruud van Nistelrooy can't hide his delight after scoring at Stamford Bridge

MANCHESTER UNITED 2

1. Fabien BARTHEZ
2. Gary NEVILLE
27. Mikael SILVESTRE
4. Juan Sebastian VERON
24. Wesley BROWN
6. Laurent BLANC
18. Paul SCHOLES
8. Nicky BUTT
20. Ole Gunnar SOLSKJAER
10. Ruud VAN NISTELROOY
11. Ryan GIGGS

SUBSTITUTES

3. Denis IRWIN (12) 88
12. Phil NEVILLE (2) 18
13. Roy CARROLL
16. Roy KEANE (18) 82
21. Diego FORLAN
28. Michael STEWART
30. John O'SHEA

ZIVKOVIC (o.g.) 29
VAN NISTELROOY (pen.) 67

MATCH REPORT

Off-key performance, disappointing result, yet another serious injury: that was the dismal story for the Red Devils as they twice surrendered the lead to the Bundesliga leaders, who left Old Trafford as firm favourites to reach the Champions League final.

The latest casualty was Gary Neville, who suffered a broken foot in an innocent challenge with Ze Roberto, though Roy Keane lit a beacon of hope for the second leg by returning ahead of schedule following his strained hamstring. United looked tense as they faced their biggest night of the season to date, and Bayer played the more fluent football throughout, yet it was the hosts who created the early opportunities.

Uncharacteristically, though, van Nistelrooy missed twice and Solskjaer shaved a post before the excellent Scholes crafted the opener with a glorious delivery to the right flank, which enabled the Dutchman to find the Norwegian, whose miscue squirmed into the net via the chest of Zivkovic.

Soon the Germans should have levelled but Berbatov shaved a post with a free header, and before half-time Silvestre at one end and Basturk at the other each went close after slaloming runs.

Bayer continued to impress in the second half and equalised deservedly through Ballack's sharp volley from Schneider's centre, but the Reds

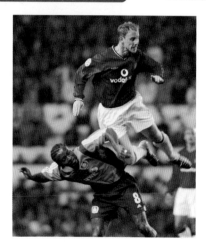

Nicky Butt rises to win the ball from Leverkusen's Ze Roberto

2 BAYER 04 LEVERKUSEN

62 BALLACK
75 NEUVILLE

1. Jorg BUTT
28. Carsten RAMELOW
35. Diego Rodolfo PLACENTE
19. LUCIO
5. Jens NOWOTNY
6. Boris ZIVKOVIC
25. Bernd SCHNEIDER
8. ZE ROBERTO
12. Dimitar BERBATOV
10. Yildiray BASTURK
13. Michael BALLACK
SUBSTITUTES
3. Marko BABIC
9. Ulf KIRSTEN
15. Jurica VRANJES (10) 78
20. Frank JURIC
26. Zoltan SEBESCEN (h-t)
27. Oliver NEUVILLE (12) 72
47. Thomas KLEINE

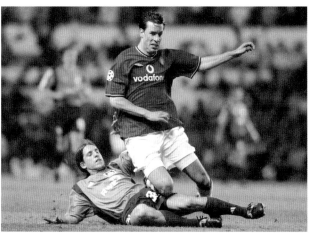

*There's no way through for Ruud van Nistelrooy as he is tackled by
defender Diego Placente*

regained the ascendancy when Veron passed sweetly to van
Nistelrooy, who was felled in the area by Ze Roberto. The
Dutchman powered in a picture-book penalty, equalling the ten-
goal record for a Champions League campaign in the process,
and the hosts seemed to be poised for victory.

But Bayer keeper Butt prevented what might have been a
decisive third goal with a flying save from Veron, who had been
set up deliciously by Giggs, then the resilient Germans
swarmed forward and Neuville tilted the tie their way by netting
after a goalmouth scramble. Suddenly the trip to Leverkusen
looked daunting indeed.

IPSWICH TOWN   0

1. Andy MARSHALL
19. Titus BRAMBLE
3. Jamie CLAPHAM
4. John McGREAL
5. Hermann HREIDARSSON
22. Tommy MILLER
33. Finidi GEORGE
8. Matt HOLLAND
38. Marcus BENT
35. Sixto PERALTA
30. Martijn REUSER

SUBSTITUTES

2. Fabian WILNIS (33) h-t
10. Alun ARMSTRONG (38) 85
11. Marcus STEWART
13. Mike SALMON
18. Darren BENT (30) 70

MATCH REPORT

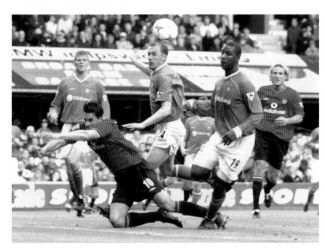

Ruud van Nistelrooy goes down between John McGreal and Titus Bramble. The result was a penalty which the Dutchman converted himself

A highly debatable penalty, earned and converted by Ruud van Nistelrooy, preserved the Red Devils' interest in the title race and left Ipswich teetering on the brink of relegation. United fielded a substantially under-strength side, but were fortified immeasurably by Roy Keane's first start since his recent hamstring injury. The skipper slipped back immediately into his most majestic form, dominating what was initially a good contest.

Both teams passed the ball fluently and there had been half-chances at either end before United began to assume command.

1 MANCHESTER UNITED

45 VAN NISTELROOY (pen.)

13. Roy CARROLL
12. Phil NEVILLE
3. Denis IRWIN
16. Roy KEANE
24. Wesley BROWN
30. John O'SHEA
28. Michael STEWART
8. Nicky BUTT
21. Diego FORLAN
10. Ruud VAN NISTELROOY
15. Luke CHADWICK
SUBSTITUTES
17. Raimond VAN DER GOUW
18. Paul SCHOLES (28) h-t
20. Ole Gunnar SOLSKJAER (10) 60
27. Mikael SILVESTRE (15) 79
32. Bojan DJORDJIC

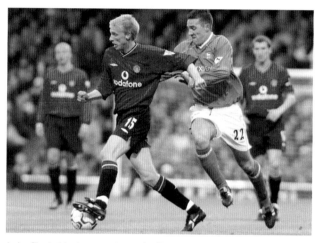

Luke Chadwick shows a clean pair of heels to Ipswich's Tommy Miller

The breakthrough came in the second minute of first-half injury time when Keane dispatched a high cross from the right and the chasing van Nistelrooy appeared to stumble between Bramble and McGreal. A penalty was awarded and the Dutchman netted unstoppably, low to Marshall's right.

Ipswich showed spirit at the outset of the second period, but soon Marshall was forced to save from Forlan (twice) and Irwin, and Keane shivered the crossbar with a sudden 30-yard scorcher. The hosts' only threat came when Peralta found Miller, whose cross-shot cleared the far post.

Thus the bitterly contested penalty had proved decisive.

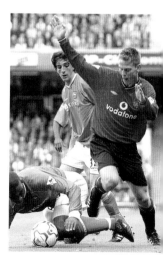

Michael Stewart made a rare start in the United line-up

BAYER 04 LEVERKUSEN 1

1. Jorg BUTT

28. Carsten RAMELOW

35. Diego Rodolfo PLACENTE

19. LUCIO

5. Jens NOWOTNY

6. Boris ZIVKOVIC

25. Bernd SCHNEIDER

8. ZE ROBERTO

27. Oliver NEUVILLE

10. Yildiray BASTURK

13. Michael BALLACK

SUBSTITUTES

3. Marko BABIC

9. Ulf KIRSTEN

12. Dimitar BERBATOV (27) 85

15. Jurica VRANJES (10) 79

20. Frank JURIC

26. Zoltan SEBESCEN (5) 10

47. Thomas KLEINE

NEUVILLE 45

Bayer Leverkusen won on away goals

MATCH REPORT

Not this time. Despite a frantic late onslaught during which they went agonisingly close to forcing victory, the luckless Red Devils mislaid their ticket to Glasgow, losing the sixth of their eight European Cup semi-finals. In all honesty, over the two legs Bayer Leverkusen deserved to win, and what pained most United fans even more than defeat itself was the fact that their multi-talented team never did themselves justice.

The Germans, a comparatively small club who have never been champions in their own land, dominated the opening exchanges and nearly went ahead after 13 minutes when

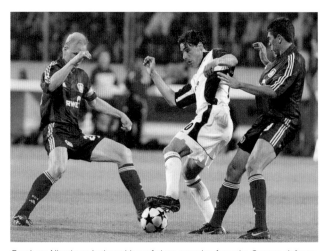

Ruud van Nistelrooy is the subject of close attention from the German defence

1 MANCHESTER UNITED

28 KEANE

1. Fabien BARTHEZ
24. Wesley BROWN
27. Mikael SILVESTRE
4. Juan Sebastian VERON
5. Ronny JOHNSEN
6. Laurent BLANC
18. Paul SCHOLES
8. Nicky BUTT
16. Roy KEANE
10. Ruud VAN NISTELROOY
11. Ryan GIGGS

SUBSTITUTES

3. Denis IRWIN (5) 60
12. Phil NEVILLE
13. Roy CARROLL
20. Ole Gunnar SOLSKJAER (8) 61
21. Diego FORLAN (24) 81
25. Quinton FORTUNE
30. John O'SHEA

Schneider beat Barthez but hit the post. However, it was United who took the lead – albeit against the run of play – when Keane exchanged passes with van Nistelrooy, then sidestepped keeper Butt and dinked home with the utmost composure from a narrow angle. That heralded a more productive interlude and both Veron and Johnsen saw goal-bound efforts diverted before Neuville equalised on the stroke of half-time, shooting in from 18 yards via the crossbar after Johnsen had slipped.

Most of the second period was scrappy, with the Reds unable to produce their characteristic sweet-passing rhythm. But hope was revived by a belated improvement which followed the arrival from the bench of Solskjaer and Forlan. However, Scholes skied from a Giggs cross, a venomous Keane drive brought a plunging save from Butt, Forlan's magnificently adroit 25-yard volley was headed off his line by Placente and Solskjaer shot marginally high.

Thus Sir Alex Ferguson's dream of lifting Europe's top club prize in his home city ended in bitter anti-climax. Perhaps next year, when the final venue is... Old Trafford.

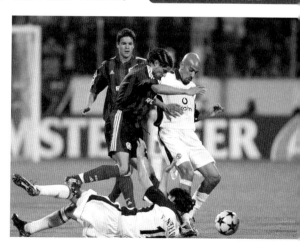

Juan Sebastian Veron fights for possession in a crowded midfield

APRIL IN REVIEW

TUESDAY 2	v DEPORTIVO LA CORUÑA	A	2-0
SATURDAY 6	v LEICESTER CITY	A	1-0
WEDNESDAY 10	v DEPORTIVO LA CORUÑA	H	3-2
SATURDAY 20	v CHELSEA	A	3-0
WEDNESDAY 24	v BAYER 04 LEVERKUSEN	H	2-2
SATURDAY 27	v IPSWICH TOWN	A	1-0
TUESDAY 30	v BAYER 04 LEVERKUSEN	A	1-1

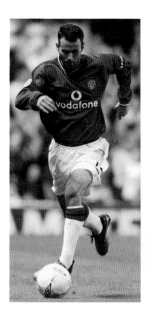

PLAYER IN THE FRAME

Ryan Giggs

Although he was effectively nullified by the close attentions of his German markers on that anti-climactic night in Leverkusen, Ryan had entertained royally earlier in the month. In both legs of the Champions League quarter-final against Deportivo he had been utterly enchanting and at Stamford Bridge he had played a telling part in all three strikes.

FA BARCLAYCARD PREMIERSHIP

UP TO AND INCLUDING
WEDNESDAY 1 MAY 2002

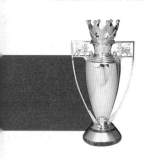

	P	W	D	L	F	A	Pts
Arsenal	36	24	9	3	74	33	81
MANCHESTER UNITED	36	24	4	8	87	44	76
Liverpool	36	22	8	6	58	27	74
Newcastle United	37	21	8	8	73	49	71
Chelsea	37	17	13	7	65	35	64
Leeds United	37	17	12	8	52	37	63
Tottenham Hotspur	37	14	8	15	48	51	50
West Ham United	37	14	8	15	46	56	50
Aston Villa	37	11	14	12	43	46	47
Middlesbrough	37	12	9	16	35	46	45
Fulham	37	10	14	13	36	41	44
Blackburn Rovers	36	11	10	15	49	47	43
Everton	37	11	10	16	42	53	43
Charlton Athletic	37	10	13	14	38	49	43
Southampton	37	11	9	17	43	53	42
Bolton Wanderers	37	9	13	15	43	60	40
Sunderland	37	10	9	18	28	50	39
Ipswich Town	37	9	9	19	41	59	36
Derby County	37	8	5	24	32	62	29
Leicester City	37	4	13	20	28	63	25

MAY

WEDNESDAY 8	**v ARSENAL**	**H**
SATURDAY 11	**v CHARLTON ATHLETIC**	**H**

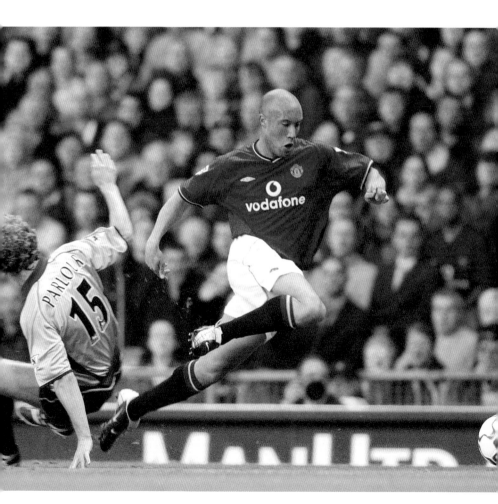

MANCHESTER UNITED 0

1. Fabien BARTHEZ
12. Phil NEVILLE
27. Mikael SILVESTRE
4. Juan Sebastian VERON
24. Wesley BROWN
6. Laurent BLANC
18. Paul SCHOLES
16. Roy KEANE
20. Ole Gunnar SOLSKJAER
21. Diego FORLAN
11. Ryan GIGGS

SUBSTITUTES

10. Ruud VAN NISTELROOY (4) 58
13. Roy CARROLL
22. Ronnie WALLWORK
25. Quinton FORTUNE (21) 69
30. John O'SHEA

MATCH REPORT

It was the stuff of nightmares. Manchester United surrendered their Premiership title to Arsenal in front of a mortified Old Trafford multitude, but in the end there could be no complaint. The Gunners, who had not lost all season on their League travels and had scored in every game, emerged as worthy victors from a contest in which the Red Devils had dominated possession, but in which they had never posed a coherent threat.

Rather misleadingly, the opening salvo was fired by the visitors as early as the second minute when Parlour broke down the right and crossed to Wiltord, whose shot was blocked by

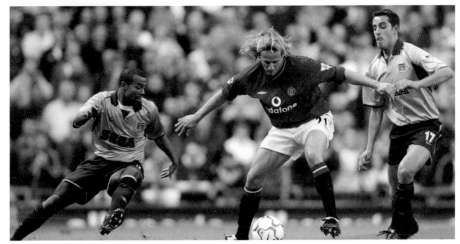

Diego Forlan dances between Ashley Cole and Edu

1 ARSENAL

56 WILTORD

1. David SEAMAN
12. LAUREN
3. Ashley COLE
4. Patrick VIEIRA
5. Martin KEOWN
23. Sol CAMPBELL
17. Ray PARLOUR
8. Fredrik LJUNGBERG
25. KANU
17. EDU
11. Sylvain WILTORD

SUBSTITUTES

2. Lee DIXON (25) 89
9. Francis JEFFERS
10. Dennis BERGKAMP
24. Richard WRIGHT
26. Igors STEPANOVS

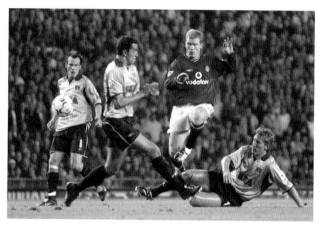

Paul Scholes gets his shot away, but the ball was diverted for a corner

Blanc. It was to be Arsenal's only meaningful attack of the half as United poured forward relentlessly. But in truth, the hosts never went closer than in the sixth minute when, after a Scholes drive was diverted for a corner, Veron crossed towards Brown and there was a shout for handball against Vieira.

Soon after the interval the decisive goal was conceded in horribly sloppy fashion. After a Silvestre slip in midfield, the ball was ferried to Ljungberg, who slipped past Blanc and shot across goal; Barthez could only parry to the unmarked Wiltord, who netted with ease. A comeback never looked likely and the arrival of van Nistelrooy from the bench made little difference. Gradually the north Londoners tightened their stranglehold on the match, and with it the Championship.

MANCHESTER UNITED 0

1. Fabien BARTHEZ

12. Phil NEVILLE

3. Denis IRWIN

28. Michael STEWART

24. Wesley BROWN

6. Laurent BLANC

18. Paul SCHOLES

16. Roy KEANE

20. Ole Gunnar SOLSKJAER

21. Diego FORLAN

25. Quinton FORTUNE

SUBSTITUTES

11. Ryan GIGGS (28) 59

17. Raimond VAN DER GOUW (1) 77

22. Ronnie WALLWORK

30. John O'SHEA (3) 69

38. Mark LYNCH

MATCH REPORT

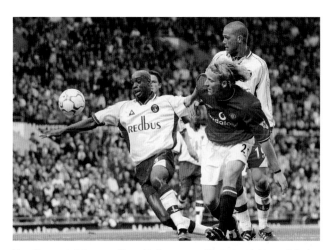

Despite several chances Diego Forlan was unable to break his goal duck

United fans craving a little light relief following recent setbacks were sorely disappointed by a frustrating stalemate, but it might have been worse. Charlton fashioned a succession of clear scoring opportunities in the first half and reached the interval kicking themselves for their failure to make them count.

United looked more sprightly in the second period, particularly after the introduction of Giggs, and at last there was a semblance of the Red Devils' customary free-flowing football. Twice in quick succession Forlan went close to breaking the deadlock. But it was typical of the endearingly eager

0 CHARLTON ATHLETIC

1. Dean KIELY
19. Luke YOUNG
3. Chris POWELL
4. Graham STUART
5. Richard RUFUS
27. Jorge COSTA
7. Chris BART-WILLIAMS
17. Scott PARKER
9. Jason EUELL
29. Kevin LISBIE
18. Paul KONCHESKY

SUBSTITUTES

13. Sasa ILIC
20. Claus JENSEN (4) 76
21. Jonatan JOHANSSON (18) 82
24. Jonathan FORTUNE
26. Mathias SVENSSON (29) 90

Uruguayan's rotten luck in front of goal since his arrival at Old Trafford in January that he failed to break his duck. Still, United almost claimed victory in added time, but Keane's shot was scrambled off the line by Kiely and, in all honesty, a draw was a fair result.

The most moving moments of the day were the farewells bade to old favourites Irwin and van der Gouw, who were both making their final appearances. The long-serving Irishman, who was skipper for the day, received a standing ovation when he was substituted, and the popular Dutchman was also accorded an appropriately affectionate send-off.

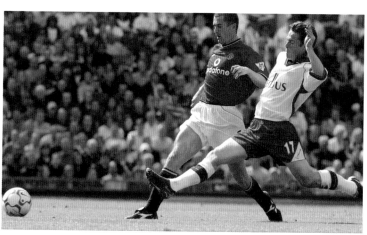

Roy Keane stretches to get the better of Charlton's Scott Parker

MAY IN REVIEW

| WEDNESDAY 8 | v ARSENAL | H | 0-1 |
| SATURDAY 11 | v CHARLTON ATHLETIC | H | 0-0 |

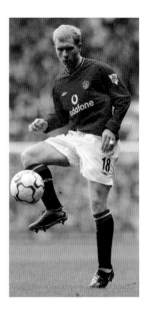

PLAYER IN THE FRAME

Paul Scholes

As Manchester United failed collectively to meet the challenge of toppling Arsenal in the Championship showdown at Old Trafford, Paul's sheer quality shone like a beacon, his dexterity on the ball matched only by the ferocity of his commitment. Though it was not his day to exercise a decisive influence, it was clear that the uncertainties of several months earlier, when a positional switch had blunted his relentless cutting edge, had been placed firmly behind him. For both United and England, that was great news.

FA BARCLAYCARD PREMIERSHIP

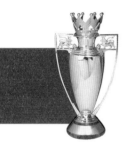

FINAL TABLE

	P	W	D	L	F	A	Pts
Arsenal	38	26	9	3	79	36	87
Liverpool	38	24	8	6	67	30	80
MANCHESTER UNITED	38	24	5	9	87	45	77
Newcastle United	38	21	8	9	74	52	71
Leeds United	38	18	12	8	53	37	66
Chelsea	38	17	13	8	66	38	64
West Ham United	38	15	8	15	48	57	53
Aston Villa	38	12	14	12	46	47	50
Tottenham Hotspur	38	14	8	16	49	53	50
Blackburn Rovers	38	12	10	16	55	51	46
Southampton	38	12	9	17	46	54	45
Middlesbrough	38	12	9	17	35	47	45
Fulham	38	10	14	14	36	44	44
Charlton Athletic	38	10	14	14	38	49	44
Everton	38	11	10	17	45	57	43
Bolton Wanderers	38	9	13	16	44	62	40
Sunderland	38	10	10	18	29	51	40
Ipswich Town	38	9	9	20	41	64	36
Derby County	38	8	6	24	33	63	30
Leicester City	38	5	13	20	30	64	28

2001–02 Season in Review

Having accepted the fact that no club can lift the League Championship every season, a look back at the 2001-02 campaign need not provoke unrelieved gloom. After all, United were trophyless for only the third time in 13 seasons, they carried the battle for the Premiership into the penultimate game, and they were just one goal away from the Champions League Final.

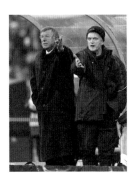

Back in early December, when Sir Alex Ferguson's men were trailing the leaders by a dozen points and every match seemed like a potential banana skin, such a comparatively lofty finish had seemed hugely improbable. Add the painful circumstance that serious injuries deprived United of Roy Keane, David Beckham and Gary Neville during the run-in, and suddenly things don't seem so bad. That said, United were defeated in no less than nine Premiership encounters – including six at Old Trafford – and that represents nearly a quarter of the programme, so there can be no complaints that the title slipped away to Arsenal, who were undeniably worthy winners.

It was always going to be a challenging term, what with the manager having announced that he would retire at its end, and with the need to integrate several new players into the side. After an encouraging start, the Reds foundered in late autumn and the vultures gathered. Fergie's footballing obituary was written, but predictions of the fearsomely driven Scot's demise proved more than a tad premature.

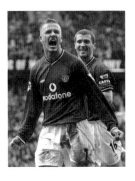

Yet again, he demonstrated stern mettle. Laying down the law to his players, demanding that they return to basics and eliminate costly individual defensive errors, he then presided over a free-scoring midwinter revival which saw them soar to the Premiership summit, and finally he changed his mind about leaving and signed a new three-year contract.

At one point a fourth successive title seemed possible, but it was not to be. Still there were some fabulous performances to savour, notably in the Champions League quarter-final clashes with Deportivo. Other mammoth pluses included 36 goals for van Nistelrooy in his debut season, 25 strikes for the wonderful Ole Gunnar Solskjaer, and encouraging progress from the youthful likes of John O'Shea and Michael Stewart.

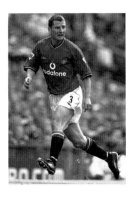

APPEARANCES

substitute appearances shown in parenthesis

	FA BARCLAYCARD PREMIERSHIP	UEFA CHAMPIONS LEAGUE	WORTHINGTON CUP	FA CUP	TOTAL
Fabien • BARTHEZ	32	15	0	1	48
Gary • NEVILLE	31 (3)	14	0	2	47 (3)
Laurent • BLANC	29	15	0	2	46
Paul • SCHOLES	30 (5)	13	0	2	45 (5)
Mikael • SILVESTRE	31 (4)	10 (3)	0	2	43 (7)
Ruud • VAN NISTELROOY	29 (3)	14	0	0 (2)	43 (5)
Roy • KEANE	28	1 (1)	0	2	41 (1)
Juan • VERON	24 (2)	13	0	1	38 (2)
David • BECKHAM	23 (5)	13	0	1	37 (5)
Ryan • GIGGS	18 (7)	13	0	0 (1)	31 (8)
Ole Gunnar • SOLSKJAER	23 (7)	5(10)	0	2	30(17)
Nicky • BUTT	20 (5)	8 (1)	0	2	30 (6)
Phil • NEVILLE	21 (7)	3 (4)	1	2	27(11)
Wesley • BROWN	15 (2)	5 (2)	0	0	20 (4)
Denis • IRWIN	10 (2)	8 (2)	0	0	18 (4)
Ronny • JOHNSEN	9 (1)	8 (1)	0	0	17 (2)
Quinton • FORTUNE	8 (6)	3 (2)	0	0	11 (8)
Roy • CARROLL	6 (1)	1	1	1	9 (1)
Andy • COLE	7 (4)	1 (3)	0	0	8 (7)
Diego • FORLAN	6 (7)	1 (4)	0	0	7(11)
Luke • CHADWICK	5 (3)	0	1	1 (1)	7 (4)
Dwight • YORKE	4 (6)	1 (2)	1	0 (1)	6 (9)
John • O'SHEA	4 (5)	0 (3)	1	0	5 (8)
Michael • STEWART	2 (1)	0 (1)	1	0	3 (2)
David • MAY	2	1	0	0	3
Ronnie • WALLWORK	0 (1)	0	1	1	2 (1)
Jimmy • DAVIS	0	0	1	0	1
Bojan • DJORDJIC	0	0	1	0	1
Lee • ROCHE	0	0	1	0	1
Jaap • STAM	1	0	0	0	1
Danny • WEBBER	0	0	1	0	1
Raimond • VAN DER GOUW	0 (1)	0	0 (1)	0	0 (2)
Michael • CLEGG	0	0	0 (1)	0	0 (1)
Daniel • NARDIELLO	0	0	0 (1)	0	0 (1)

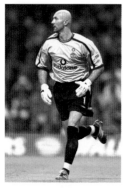

Fabien Barthez

GOALSCORERS

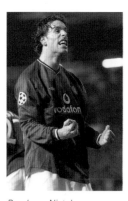

Ruud van Nistelrooy

	FA BARCLAYCARD PREMIERSHIP	UEFA CHAMPIONS LEAGUE	WORTHINGTON CUP	FA CUP	TOTAL
Ruud • VAN NISTELROOY	23	10	0	2	35
Ole Gunnar • SOLSKJAER	17	7	0	1	25
David • BECKHAM	11	5	0	0	16
Ryan • GIGGS	7	2	0	0	9
Paul • SCHOLES	8	1	0	0	9
Andy • COLE	4	1	0	0	5
Juan • VERON	5	0	0	0	5
Roy • KEANE	3	1	0	0	4
Laurent • BLANC	1	2	0	0	3
Phil • NEVILLE	2	0	0	0	2
Nicky • BUTT	1	0	0	0	1
Quinton • FORTUNE	1	0	0	0	1
Ronny • JOHNSEN	1	0	0	0	1
Mikael • SILVESTRE	0	1	0	0	1
Dwight • YORKE	1	0	0	0	1
ALPAY • Ozalan (Aston Villa)	1 o.g.	0	0	0	1 o.g.
Stanislav • VARGA (Sunderland)	1 o.g.	0	0	0	1 o.g.
Boris • ZIVKOVIC (Bayer 04)	0	1 o.g.	0	0	1 o.g.
Total	**87**	**31**	**0**	**3**	**121**

LEAGUE ATTENDANCES 2001-02

Home		Away	
67,683	v Middlesbrough	52,056	v Newcastle United
67,651	v Leicester City	48,305	v Sunderland
67,646	v Newcastle United	44,361	v Liverpool
67,638	v Southampton	42,632	v Aston Villa
67,599	v Liverpool	41,725	v Chelsea
67,599	v Tottenham Hotspur	40,058	v Leeds United
67,592	v Aston Villa	39,948	v Everton
67,587	v Sunderland	38,174	v Arsenal
67,582	v West Ham United	36,038	v Tottenham Hotspur
67,577	v Derby County	35,281	v West Ham United
67,571	v Charlton Athletic	34,358	v Middlesbrough
67,580	v Arsenal	33,041	v Derby County
67,559	v Bolton Wanderers	31,858	v Southampton
67,555	v Leeds United	29,836	v Blackburn Rovers
67,552	v Blackburn Rovers	28,433	v Ipswich Town
67,551	v Ipswich Town	27,350	v Bolton Wanderers
67,544	v Chelsea	26,475	v Charlton Athletic
67,534	v Everton	21,447	v Leicester City
67,534	v Fulham	21,159	v Fulham

Home		Away	
Highest	v 67,683 (Middlesbrough)	Highest	v 52,056 (Newcastle United)
Lowest	v 67,534 (Everton, Fulham)	Lowest	v 21,159 (Fulham)
Total	1,284,134	Total	672,535
Average	67,586	Average	35,396

OLD TRAFFORD ATTENDANCES

League & Cup

Total   1,813,308

Average   67,159

Includes: 19 FA Carling Premiership games

8 UEFA Champions League games

Sunday 12 August, 2001 • Millennium Stadium, Cardiff • 2.00pm • Attendance 70,227
Referee Andy D'Urso

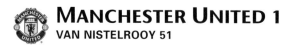

MANCHESTER UNITED 1
VAN NISTELROOY 51

LIVERPOOL 2
McALLISTER 2 (pen.)
OWEN 16

MATCH REPORT

Another year, another Charity Shield defeat, but there was a marked absence of Mancunian despair at the end of 90 entertaining minutes under Cardiff's most capacious roof. After all, the Red Devils had kicked off each of the three previous campaigns by losing this friendly opener, then gone on to win the Premiership title. That said, this was the third successive defeat by Liverpool and although Sir Alex Ferguson's men held their own in the game – dominating the second half after a wan display for most of the first – the sight of silverware headed for Merseyside was hardly a welcome climax to his side's first visit to the Millennium.

United could not have made a more inauspicious beginning. Barely a minute had passed when Owen crossed to Murphy, who had nudged the ball out of immediate danger when Keane brought him down in the box. McAllister sent Barthez the wrong way from the spot and the Scouse legions howled their glee. Soon worse was to follow as Stam slipped when attempting to reach Westerveld's raking punt and the ball fell to Owen, who dodged Neville before shooting neatly past Barthez.

Gradually the Red Devils rallied as the interval approached. A Keane header forced a brilliant save from Westerveld, Henchoz handballed Silvestre's drive but no penalty was awarded, then Keane cracked the Liverpool crossbar from 25 yards. The second half was

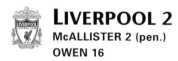

MANCHESTER UNITED 1 Fabien BARTHEZ, 2 Gary NEVILLE, 3 Denis IRWIN, 16 Roy KEANE, 27 Mikael SILVESTRE, 6 Jaap STAM, 7 David BECKHAM, 8 Nicky BUTT, 18 Paul SCHOLES, 10 Ruud VAN NISTELROOY, 11 Ryan GIGGS **Substitutes:** 5 Ronny JOHNSEN, 12 Phil NEVILLE 13 Roy CARROLL, 15 Luke CHADWICK, 19 Dwight YORKE (8) 66, 20 Ole Gunnar SOLSKJAER, 24 Wesley BROWN

LIVERPOOL 1 Sander WESTERVELD, 2 Stephane HENCHOZ, 18 John Arne RIISE, 4 Sami HYYPIA, 16 Dietmar HAMANN 6 Markus BABBEL, 20 Nick BARMBY, 8 Emile HESKEY, 21 Gary McALLISTER, 10 Michael OWEN, 13 Danny MURPHY **Substitutes:** 11 Jamie REDKNAPP, 15 Patrik BERGER (13) 72, 19 Pegguy ARPHEXAD, 23 Jamie CARRAGHER (18) 84, 25 Igor BISCAN (20) 72, 30 Djimi TRAORE, 37 Jari LITMANEN

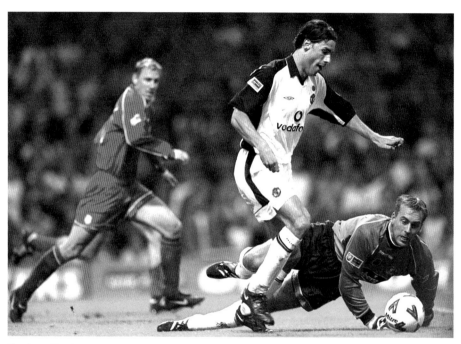

Ruud van Nistelrooy guides the ball carefully past Westerveld to score his first goal for United...

all United and debutant van Nistelrooy had already missed two clear openings when he pounced on a Giggs pass, sidestepped Westerveld and netted with alacrity, a slick finish which promised riches to come.

Thereafter the champions launched a blitz during which Beckham, Scholes, Keane, Neville, and van Nistelrooy all went close, but they were foiled by the athleticism of Westerveld and another negative response from the referee following a second Henchoz handball.

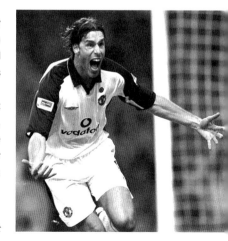

... and clearly registers his delight

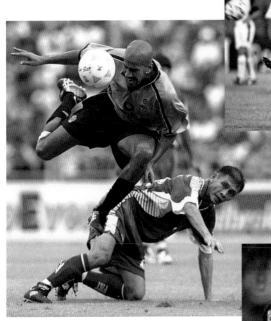

Action from all three of United's matches on the pre-season trip to Asia in July 2001

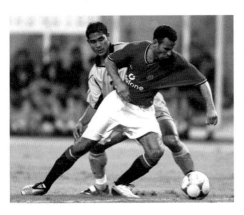

names in bold indicate goalscorers

v MALAYSIA ALL-STARS (Bukit Jalil Stadium, Kuala Lumpur) • Attendance: 100,000 • Won: 6-0
Sunday 22 July 2001

Barthez • Neville G. • Irwin • Veron • Johnsen • Stam • **Beckham** • Keane • Yorke • **van Nistelrooy 2** • Giggs
Substitutes: Neville P. (Irwin) • *van der Gouw* • *Brown (Johnsen)* • ***Chadwick** (Beckham)* • *Butt (Keane)* •
***Cole 2** (Yorke)* • *Scholes (Veron)* • *Fortune (Giggs)* • *Solskjaer (van Nistelrooy)*

v TEAM SINGAPORE (Kallang Stadium, Singapore) • Attendance: 44,000 • Won: 8-1
Tuesday 24 July 2001

van der Gouw • Neville G. • **Neville P.** • Veron • Brown • Stam • **Beckham** • Keane • **Solskjaer 2** • **van Nistelrooy** • Scholes
Substitutes: Silvestre (Neville P.) • *Barthez (van Nistelrooy)* • *Irwin (Stam)* • ***Yorke 2** (Solskjaer)* • *Fortune (Beckham)* •
Chadwick (Veron) • ***Giggs** (Keane)*

v THAILAND (Rajamangala Stadium, Bangkok) • Attendance: 65,000 • Won: 2-1
Sunday 29 July 2001

Barthez • Brown • Irwin • Veron • Johnsen • Silvestre • Beckham • Butt • Cole • van Nistelrooy • **Giggs**
Substitutes: Neville P. (Irwin) • *van der Gouw (Barthez)* • *Stam* • *Neville G. (Cole)* • *Keane (Veron)* • *Fortune (Giggs)* •
Scholes (Butt) • ***Yorke** (van Nistelrooy)* • *Chadwick (Beckham)*

v CELTIC (home) • Attendance: 66,957 • Lost: 3-4
Wednesday 1 August 2001

Barthez • Neville G. • Irwin • **Veron** • Neville P. • Stam • Beckham • Scholes • Keane • **van Nistelrooy 2** • Giggs
Substitutes: Johnsen (Neville G.) • *Cantona (Scholes)* • *Butt (Keane)* • *Cole* • *van der Gouw* • *Brown (Irwin)* • *Chadwick (Veron)* •
Silvestre (Neville P.) • *Yorke (Beckham)* • *Solskjaer*

v WREXHAM (away) • Attendance: 7,614 • Drew: 2-2
Saturday 4 August 2001

Carroll • Neville G. • Silvestre • **Veron** • May • Stam • Chadwick • Scholes • **Solskjaer** • van Nistelrooy • Giggs
Substitutes: Wallwork (Neville G.) • *Rachubka (Carroll)* • *O'Shea (Stam)* • *Nardiello (van Nistelrooy)* • *Davis (Scholes)* •
Rankin (Solskjaer) • *Williams M. (Chadwick)* • *Muirhead (Giggs)*

v BURY (away) • Attendance: 9,929 • Won: 3-0
Wednesday 8 August 2001

van der Gouw • Neville G. • **Neville P.** • Brown • Silvestre • **Yorke** • Chadwick • Butt • Cole • **Solskjaer** • Fortune
Substitutes: May (Neville G.) • *Carroll (van der Gouw)* • *Roche (Neville P.)* • *O'Shea (Silvestre)* • *Djordjic (Fortune)* •
Stewart (Chadwick) • *Wallwork (Butt)*

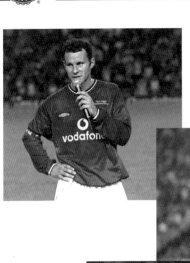

A selection of pictures taken at Ryan Giggs's testimonial match against Celtic at Old Trafford on 1 August 2001 which included the return of Eric Cantona and a brace of goals for new-boy Ruud van Nistelrooy

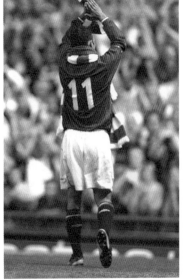

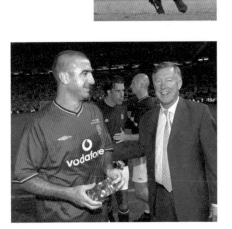

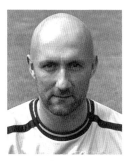

FABIEN BARTHEZ

Position: goalkeeper
Born: Lavelanet, France, 28 June 1971
Transferred: from AS Monaco, 21 May 2000
Other clubs: Toulouse, Olympique Marseille, AS Monaco
Senior United debut: 13 August 2000 v Chelsea at Wembley
(FA Charity Shield)
United record: League: 62 games, 0 goals; FA Cup: 2 games,
0 goals; League Cup: 0 games, 0 goals; Europe: 27 games,
0 goals; Others: 2 games, 0 goals
Total: 93 games, 0 goals
Full International: France
In 2001-02: Fabien did not maintain the impeccable level of consistency which he achieved
in his first season in England, yet still he shone as one of the Premiership's most
accomplished goalkeepers. True, there were some costly high-profile mistakes, but
invariably they were mitigated by the charismatic Frenchman's brilliance in the same
match, for example against Arsenal at Highbury.

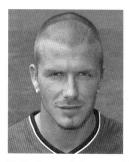

DAVID BECKHAM

Position: midfielder
Born: Leytonstone, 2 May 1975
Signed trainee: 8 July 1991
Signed professional: 23 January 1993
Other club: Preston North End (loan)
Senior United debut: 23 September 1992 v Brighton & Hove
Albion at the Goldstone Ground (League Cup, substitute for
Andrei Kanchelskis)
United record: League: 210 (24) games, 56 goals; FA Cup: 19 (2) games, 5 goals; League
Cup: 5 (2) games, 0 goals; Europe: 69 (2) games, 12 goals; Others: 8 (2) games, 1 goal
Total: 311 (32) games, 74 goals
Full international: England
In 2001-02: England's captain experienced a season of highs and lows. There were interludes
when he touched his majestic best and his 16 goals for United – including sensational efforts at
West Ham and in La Coruña – represented his highest-ever tally. Against that there was a
serious lapse of form in mid-season and a broken foot which sidelined him during the spring.

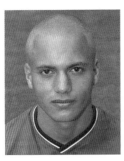

WESLEY BROWN

Position: defender
Born: Manchester, 13 October 1979
Signed trainee: 8 July 1996
Signed professional: 4 November 1996
Senior United debut: 4 May 1998 v Leeds United at Old Trafford
(League, substitute for David May)
United record: League: 52 (9) games, 0 goals; FA Cup: 3 games,
0 goals; League Cup: 1 (1) games, 0 goals; Europe: 17 (5) games,
0 goals; Others: 0 games, 0 goals
Total: 73 (15) games, 0 goals
Full international: England
In 2001-02: Wes was given an early chance to consolidate his place following the departure of Jaap Stam, but his progress was hindered by injuries which sidelined him from December until April. This was chronic luck for a richly promising youngster whose early career has been plagued abominably by fitness problems, but he fought back courageously to earn a berth in England's World Cup squad.

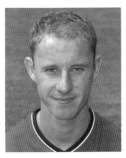

NICKY BUTT

Position: midfielder
Born: Manchester, 21 January 1975
Signed trainee: 8 July 1991
Signed professional: 23 January 1993
Senior United debut: 21 November 1992 v Oldham Athletic at
Old Trafford (League, substitute for Paul Ince)
United record: League: 184 (47) games, 20 goals; FA Cup: 20 (2)
games, 1 goal; League Cup: 5 games, 0 goals; Europe: 46 (12)
games, 2 goals; Others: 8 games, 2 goals
Total: 263 (61) games, 25 goals
Full international: England
In 2001-02: Nicky offered further evidence – as if it were needed – that he is a massive asset to Manchester United, a performer whose all-round game has matured noticeably. After the side had struggled dismally in the autumn, he was drafted into central midfield and excelled alongside Roy Keane, his insatiable spirit and work-rate proving hugely instrumental in the subsequent revival.

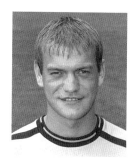

ROY CARROLL

Position: goalkeeper
Born: Enniskillen, Northern Ireland, 30 September 1977
Transferred: from Wigan Athletic
Other clubs: Hull City, Wigan Athletic
Senior United debut: 26 August 2001 v Aston Villa at Villa Park (League)
United record: League: 6 (1) games, 0 goals; FA Cup: 1 game, 0 goals; League Cup: 1 game, 0 goals; Europe: 1 game, 0 goals; Others: 0 games, 0 goals
Total: 9 (1) games, 0 goals
In 2001-02: Roy created a splendid impression during his first campaign in the top flight. Succeeding Raimond van der Gouw as chief understudy to Fabien Barthez, he displayed lithe athleticism, a safe pair of hands, a shrewd positional sense and admirable composure, no matter how pressurised the situation. The tall Ulsterman appears to have all the makings of a front-rank keeper.

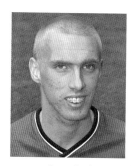

LUKE CHADWICK

Position: forward
Born: Cambridge, 18 November 1980
Signed trainee: 30 June 1997
Signed professional: 5 February 1999
Other club: Royal Antwerp (loan)
Senior United debut: 13 October 1999 v Aston Villa at Villa Park (League Cup)
United record: League: 11 (13) games, 2 goals; FA Cup: 1 (2) games, 0 goals; League Cup: 4 games, 0 goals; Europe: 1 (2) games, 0 goals; Others: 0 games, 0 goals
Total: 17 (17) game, 2 goals
In 2001-02: Having demonstrated his worth during the previous campaign as a penetrating raider who can thrive on either wing, Luke set the pulses racing with scintillating autumn displays at home to Everton and against Sunderland at the Stadium of Light. Later, though, his impetus was interrupted by a hernia operation and he did not return to the first-team reckoning until late spring.

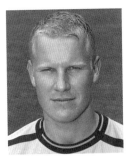

NICK CULKIN

Position: goalkeeper
Born: York, 6 July 1978
Transferred: from York City, 25 September 1995
Other clubs: York City, Hull City (loan), Bristol Rovers (loan), Livingston (loan)
Senior United debut: 22 August 1999 v Arsenal at Highbury (League, substitute for Raimond van der Gouw)
United record: League: 0 (1) games, 0 goals; FA Cup: 0 games, 0 goals; League Cup: 0 games, 0 goals; Europe: 0 games, 0 goals; Others: 0 games, 0 goals
Total: 0 (1) games, 0 goals
In 2001-02: Nick became an unfamiliar figure at Old Trafford, spending most of the campaign north of the border, where his consistent displays between Livingston's posts helped the Lions to finish third in their initial term among the Scottish elite. It was the second successive season the big, blond custodian had spent almost entirely on loan, having served Bristol Rovers in 2000-2001.

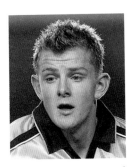

JIMMY DAVIS

Position: forward
Born: Bromsgrove, 6 February 1982
Signed trainee: 6 July 1999
Signed professional: 31 August 1999
Senior United debut: 5 November 2001 v Arsenal at Highbury (League Cup)
United record: League: 0 games, 0 goals; FA Cup: 0 games, 0 goals; League Cup: 1 game, 0 goals; Europe: 0 games, 0 goals; Others: 0 games, 0 goals
Total: 1 game, 0 goals
In 2001-02: Jimmy continued his rise through the Red Devils junior ranks alongside his contemporary, fellow marksman Danny Webber. A spirited raider who can also operate on the right flank, he featured regularly for the reserves, contributing admirably to the lifting of the Premiership Reserve League (North) title, and performed promisingly for England at under-20 level.

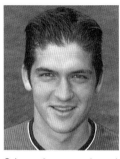

BOJAN DJORDJIC

Position: midfielder
Born: Belgrade, Yugoslavia, 6 February 1982
Transferred from: Brommapojkarna IF, 17 February 1999
Other clubs: Brommapojkarna IF, Sheffield Wednesday (loan)
Senior United debut: 19 May 2001 v Tottenham Hotspur at
White Hart Lane (League, substitute for Denis Irwin)
United record: League: 0 (1) games, 0 goals; FA Cup: 0 games,
0 goals; League Cup: 1 game, 0 goals; Europe: 0 games, 0 goals;
Others: 0 games, 0 goals
Total: 1 (1) games, 0 goals
In 2001-02: Bojan completed a fruitful season with the reserves, his clever work on the left side of midfield taking the eye, along with his accomplishment in dead-ball situations. The Swedish under-21 international excelled, too, during a brief loan stint with Sheffield Wednesday and further progress might see him knocking at the door of the Red Devils' senior squad in 2002-03.

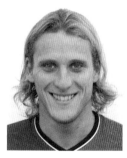

DIEGO FORLAN

Position: forward
Born: Montevideo, Uruguay, 19 May 1979
Transferred: from Independiente
Other clubs: Independiente   2 0 0 2
Senior United debut: 29 January 2001 v Bolton Wanderers at the
Reebok Stadium (League, substitute for Ole Gunnar Solskjaer)
United record: League: 6 (7) games, 0 goals; FA Cup: 0 games,
0 goals; League Cup: 0 games, 0 goals; Europe: 1 (4) games,
0 goals; Others: 0 games, 0 goals
Total: 7 (11) games, 0 goals
Full international: Uruguay
In 2001-02: Diego strove manfully to adapt to the English game but, not surprisingly for a relatively inexperienced South American, he did not find it easy. Though everyone at Old Trafford was willing him to break his scoring duck, that crucial first goal proved frustratingly elusive. However, his pace, deft touch and endless enthusiasm augured favourably for a productive future.

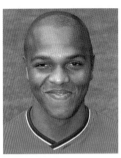

QUINTON FORTUNE

Position: forward or midfielder
Born: Cape Town, South Africa, 21 May 1977
Transferred: from Atletico Madrid, 21 August 1999
Other club: Atletico Madrid
Senior United debut: 30 August 1999 v Newcastle United at
Old Trafford (League, substitute for Paul Scholes)
United record: League: 18 (9) games, 5 goals; FA Cup: 0 games,
0 goals; League Cup: 2 games, 0 goals; Europe: 4 (6) games,
0 goals; Others: 1 (2) games, 2 goals
Total: 25 (17) games, 7 goals
Full international: South Africa
In 2001-02: Quinton offered decent cover as a wide midfielder, looking particularly effective
as a deputy for Ryan Giggs in the early part of the season. Thereafter his contribution was
limited by his participation in the African Nations Cup, but a few more outings followed in
the spring and the strong, hard-running South African never let the Red Devils down.

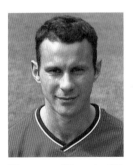

RYAN GIGGS

Position: forward
Born: Cardiff, 29 November 1973
Signed trainee: 9 July 1990
Signed professional: 29 November 1990
Senior United debut: 2 March 1991 v Everton at Old Trafford
(League, substitute for Denis Irwin)
United record: League: 309 (37) games, 71 goals; FA Cup: 36 (4)
games, 7 goals; League Cup: 17 (4) games, 6 goals; Europe: 64
(3) games, 15 goals; Others: 10 (1) games, 0 goals
Total: 436 (49) games, 99 goals
Full international: Wales
In 2001-02: For much of the campaign Ryan melded brilliance with consistency and tore many
a defence to shreds with his unpredictable high-speed runs, whether starting from his
customary left-flank position or as a slightly withdrawn front-man. He was sorely missed when
sidelined by hamstring trouble in the autumn, and later he was a popular choice as captain in
Keane's absence.

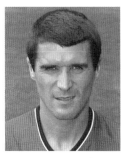

ROY KEANE

Position: midfielder
Born: Cork, 10 August 1971
Transferred: from Nottingham Forest, 19 July 1993
Other clubs: Cobh Ramblers, Nottingham Forest
Senior United debut: 15 August 1993 v Norwich City at Carrow Road (League)
United record: League: 233 (8) games, 29 goals; FA Cup: 33 (1) games, 1 goal; League Cup: 9 (2) games, 0 goals; Europe: 64 (1) games, 15 goals; Others: 10 games, 2 goals
Total: 349 (12) games, 47 goals
Full international: Republic of Ireland
In 2001-02: Roy continued to be the most influential of all current Red Devils, and United never looked quite the same force during his absences with knee and hamstring injuries. The inspirational skipper is magnificent in every aspect of play, though his immense skill and creativity are often underrated due to media preoccupation with his awesome physical and leadership qualities.

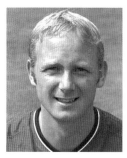

DAVID MAY

Position: defender
Born: Oldham, 24 June 1970
Transferred: from Blackburn Rovers, 1 July 1994
Other clubs: Blackburn Rovers, Huddersfield Town (loan)
Senior United debut: 14 August 1994 v Blackburn Rovers at Wembley (FA Charity Shield)
United record: League: 68 (16) games, 6 goals; FA Cup: 6 games, 0 goals; League Cup: 7 games, 1 goal; Europe: 13 (1) games, 1 goal; Others: 2 (1) games, 0 goals
Total: 96 (18) games, 8 goals
In 2001-02: Yet again David was frustrated by niggling injuries which limited his first-team involvement, though he performed solidly when making a brief return to the Champions League stage in Lille. However, he proved invaluable at reserve level, where his experience and composure set a splendid example for the youngsters around him, and his title medal was richly deserved.

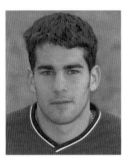

DANIEL NARDIELLO

Position: forward
Born: Coventry, 22 October 1982
Signed trainee: 5 July 1999
Signed professional: 22 October 1999
Senior United debut: 5 November 2001 v Arsenal at Highbury
(League Cup, substitute for Bojan Djordjic)
United record: League: 0 games, 0 goals; FA Cup: 0 games,
0 goals; League Cup: 0 (1) games, 0 goals; Europe: 0 games,
0 goals; Others: 0 games, 0 goals
Total: 0 (1) games, 0 goals

In 2001-02: Daniel earned his breakthrough to the senior ranks with consistent success at under-19 and reserve level. A strong, hard-running front-man, he is both a taker and maker of goals, his finishing ability being underpinned by assured control and intelligent distribution, which enables him to bring colleagues into the game. His father, Donato, was a Welsh international.

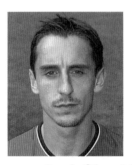

GARY NEVILLE

Position: defender
Born: Bury, 18 February 1975
Signed trainee: 8 July 1991
Signed professional: 23 January 1993
Senior United debut: 16 September 1992 v Torpedo Moscow at
Old Trafford (UEFA Cup, substitute for Lee Martin)
United record: League: 230 (7) games, 3 goals; FA Cup: 25 (3)
games, 0 goals; League Cup: 4 (1) games, 0 goals; Europe: 69 (3)
games, 0 goals; Others: 7 (1) games, 0 goals
Total: 335 (15) games, 3 goals
Full international: England

In 2001-02: Gary began impressively at right-back before an autumn dip in form. However, he bounced back with typical resilience to complete an outstanding midwinter stint in central defence, where his pace and aggression made him an ideal foil for the stately Laurent Blanc. Later he returned successfully to the flank, where he suffered the foot injury which kept him out of the World Cup.

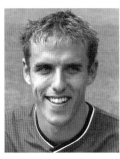

PHIL NEVILLE

Position: defender
Born: Bury, 21 January 1977
Signed trainee: 5 July 1993
Signed professional: 1 June 1994
Senior United debut: 28 January 1995 v Wrexham at Old Trafford (FA Cup)
United record: League: 150 (38) games, 4 goals; FA Cup: 17 (4) games, 0 goals; League Cup: 8 (1) games, 0 goals; Europe: 25 (15) games, 1 goal; Others: 6 (2) games, 0 goals
Total: 206 (60) games, 5 goals
Full international: England
In 2001-02: Phil struck a vein of admirably consistent form in mid-season when he was granted an extended run in the side. Settling smoothly in his natural right-back slot, he looked at ease in both defence and attack, but by springtime he was back on the bench and missed selection for England's World Cup party. Endlessly adaptable, he remains an integral part of United's squad.

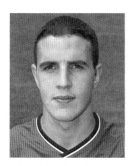

JOHN O'SHEA

Position: defender
Born: Waterford, Republic of Ireland, 30 April 1981
Signed professional: 3 August 1998
Other clubs: AFC Bournemouth (loan), Royal Antwerp (loan)
Senior United debut: 13 October 1999 v Aston Villa at Villa Park (League Cup)
United record: League: 4 (5) games, 0 goals; FA Cup: 0 games, 0 goals; League Cup: 4 games, 0 goals; Europe: 0 (3) games, 0 goal; Others: 0 games, 0 goals
Total: 8 (8) games, 0 goals
Full international: Republic of Ireland
In 2001-02: John looked to be an exceptional central defender in the making, a footballing stopper whose cultured distribution and assurance in possession would be the envy of many a midfielder. Blessed with a cool temperament, he demonstrated quality under pressure when rising from the bench in Lille, then excelled at home to Boavista and in three successive Premiership starts. One to watch.

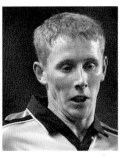

LEE ROCHE

Position: defender
Born: Bolton, 28 October 1980
Signed trainee: 30 June 1997
Signed professional: 5 February 1999
Other club: Wrexham (loan)
Senior United debut: 5 November 2001 v Arsenal at Highbury
(League Cup)
United record: League: 0 games, 0 goals; FA Cup: 0 games,
0 goals; League Cup: 1 game, 0 goals; Europe: 0 games 0 goals; Others: 0 games, 0 goals
Total: 1 game, 0 goals
In 2001-02: Lee tasted senior action with the Reds for the first time, though already he had garnered League experience, missing only a handful of Division Two outings for Wrexham during his extended loan of the previous term. This time the overlapping right-back featured regularly for United's title-winning reserves, proving solid in defence and enterprising in attack.

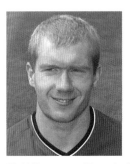

PAUL SCHOLES

Position: midfielder or forward
Born: Salford, 16 November 1974
Signed trainee: 8 July 1991
Signed professional: 23 January 1993
Senior United debut: 21 September 1994 v Port Vale at Vale Park
(League Cup)
United record: League: 175 (52) games, 55 goals; FA Cup: 10 (7)
games, 4 goals; League Cup: 6 (2) games, 5 goals; Europe:
53 (10) games, 17 goals; Others: 8 games, 0 goals
Total: 252 (71) games, 81 goals
Full international: England
In 2001-02: Paul endured a few difficult months when deployed as a deep-lying front-man, just behind Ruud van Nistelrooy. In that advanced role, perhaps, he lacked the room to express himself, but when restored to midfield he returned to prime form, even when circumstances dictated that he start on the flank. Paul remains arguably the Premiership's most consistently incisive passer.

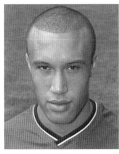

MIKAEL SILVESTRE

Position: defender
Born: Chambray-Les-Tours, France, 9 August 1977
Transferred: from Internazionale, 10 September 1999
Other clubs: Rennes, Internazionale
Senior United debut: 11 September 1999 v Liverpool at Anfield (League)
United record: League: 86 (10) games, 1 goal; FA Cup: 4 games, 0 goals; League Cup: 0 games, 0 goals; Europe: 25 (6) games, 1 goal; Others: 5 games, 0 goals
Total: 120 (16) games, 2 goals
Full international: France
In 2001-02: Mikael suffered one or two early stutters before his pace, power and improved level of concentration made the left-back berth his exclusive property. At times he surged forward dynamically and dispatched some devastating crosses, though more reliable distribution would be ideal. He displayed his prowess at centre-back, too, emerging as man of the match in Lille.

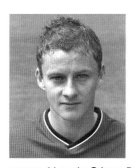

OLE GUNNAR SOLSKJAER

Position: forward
Born: Kristiansund, Norway, 26 February 1973
Transferred: from Molde, 29 July 1996
Other clubs: Clausenengen FK, Molde
Senior United debut: 25 August 1996 v Blackburn Rovers at Old Trafford (League, substitute for David May)
United record: League: 106 (57) games, 75 goals; FA Cup: 8 (9) games, 5 goals; League Cup: 6 games, 5 goals; Europe: 24 (35) games, 14 goals; Others: 5 (3) games, 0 goals
Total: 149 (104) games, 99 goals
Full international: Norway
In 2001-02: After burnishing his 'supersub' reputation with several key strikes, Ole was given a regular starting berth and responded by completing his most prolific campaign to date. Meshing potently with Ruud van Nistelrooy, he netted 25 times, plundering some of the most breathtaking goals in United's modern history. In both attitude and performance, the Norwegian is a veritable treasure.

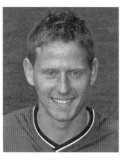

MICHAEL STEWART

Position: midfielder
Born: Edinburgh, 26 February 1981
Signed trainee: 30 June 1997
Signed professional: 13 March 1998
Senior United debut: 31 October 2000 v Watford at Vicarage Road (League Cup, substitute for Ronnie Wallwork)
United record: League: 5 (1) games, 0 goals; FA Cup: 0 games, 0 goals; League Cup: 1 (2) games, 0 goals; Europe: 0 (1) games, 0 goals; Others: 0 games, 0 goals
Total: 6 (4) games, 0 goals

In 2001-02: Michael made significant personal strides despite enjoying only a handful of senior outings, earning both his full international debut and a new four-year contract at Old Trafford. The flame-haired Scottish central midielder, who skippered the reserves to title success, is not a flashy performer, but his blend of skill, intelligence and industry bodes well for the future.

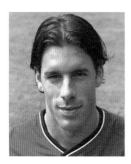

RUUD VAN NISTELROOY

Position: forward
Born: Oss, Holland, 1 July 1976
Transferred: from PSV Eindhoven, 1 July 2001
Other clubs: Den Bosch, Heerenveen, PSV Eindhoven
Senior United debut: 12 August 2001 v Liverpool at the Millennium Stadium (FA Charity Shield)
United record: League: 29 (3) games, 23 goals; FA Cup: 0 (2) games, 2 goals; League Cup: 0 games, 0 goals; Europe: 14 games, 10 goals; Others: 1 game, 1 goal
Total: 44 (5) games, 36 goals
Full international: Holland

In 2001-02: The Dutch sharp-shooter with no perceptible weakness to his game achieved success beyond all realistic expectations, scoring freely in his first English term, an astonishing feat after missing almost the whole of the previous season with an horrendous knee injury. Fittingly, he was voted player of the year by his fellow professionals, and his horizons appear limitless.

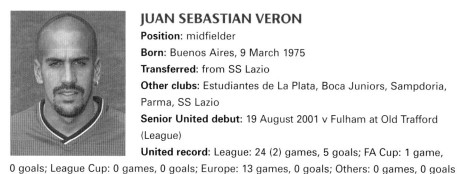

JUAN SEBASTIAN VERON

Position: midfielder
Born: Buenos Aires, 9 March 1975
Transferred: from SS Lazio
Other clubs: Estudiantes de La Plata, Boca Juniors, Sampdoria, Parma, SS Lazio
Senior United debut: 19 August 2001 v Fulham at Old Trafford (League)
United record: League: 24 (2) games, 5 goals; FA Cup: 1 game, 0 goals; League Cup: 0 games, 0 goals; Europe: 13 games, 0 goals; Others: 0 games, 0 goals
Total: 38 (2) games, 5 goals
Full international: Argentina
In 2001-02: The extravagantly gifted Argentinian play-maker made a supreme beginning to life as a Red Devil, passing like a god and netting three times in his first six Premiership starts. But, as his settling-in period progressed, his form fluctuated and he suffered heavy media flak. The manager retained faith in his record signing, however, and seldom is he proved wrong!

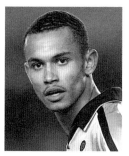

DANNY WEBBER

Position: forward
Born: Manchester, 28 December 1981
Signed trainee: 6 July 1998
Signed professional: 28 December 1998
Other clubs: Port Vale (loan), Watford (loan)
Senior United debut: 28 November 2000 v Sunderland at the Stadium of Light (League Cup, substitute for Ronnie Wallwork)
United record: League: 0 games, 0 goals; FA Cup: 0 games, 0 goals; League Cup: 1 (1) games, 0 goals; Europe: 0 games, 0 goals; Others: 0 games, 0 goals
Total: 1 (1) games, 0 goals
In 2001-02: Danny was the reserves' leading scorer and, though he was granted only one senior appearance for the Red Devils, the quick, effervescent marksman heightened his profile with successful loan spells at Port Vale and Watford. The England under-20 international shone particularly brightly at Vicarage Road, netting two League goals and plaguing several First Division defences.

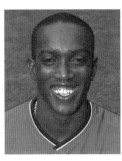

DWIGHT YORKE

Position: forward

Born: Canaan, Tobago, 3 November 1971

Transferred: from Aston Villa, 20 August 1998

Other club: Aston Villa

Senior United debut: 22 August 1998 v West Ham United at Upton Park (League)

United record: League: 80 (16) games, 48 goals; FA Cup: 6 (5) games, 3 goals; League Cup: 3 games, 2 goals; Europe: 28 (8) games, 11 goals; Others: 3 (3) games, 2 goals

Total: 120 (32) games, 66 goals

Full international: Trinidad and Tobago

In 2001-02: Dwight endured a season to forget, almost certainly his last at Old Trafford. Starting behind van Nistelrooy, Solskjaer and Cole in the strikers' pecking order, he grew frustrated with his bit-part role and was the subject of constant transfer speculation. For all that, his overall strike-rate as a Red remains magnificent and his part in the famous treble will never be forgotten.

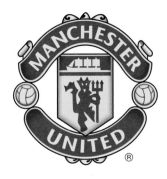

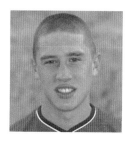

JOHN COGGER
Position: defender
Birthdate: 12 September 1983
Birthplace: Waltham Forest
Signed trainee: 3 July 2000
Signed professional: 1 July 2001

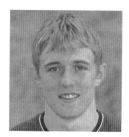

DARREN FLETCHER
Position: midfield
Birthdate: 1 February 1984
Birthplace: Edinburgh
Signed trainee: 3 July 2000
Signed professional: 1 February 2001

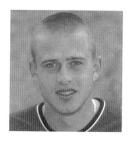

DAVID FOX
Position: midfield
Birthdate: 13 December 1983
Birthplace: Stoke-on-Trent
Signed trainee: 3 July 2000
Signed professional: 13 December 2000

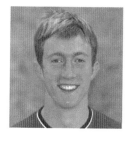

COLIN HEATH
Position: forward
Birthdate: 31 December 1983
Birthplace: Chesterfield
Signed trainee: 3 July 2000
Signed professional: 31 December 2000

PLAYER PROFILES

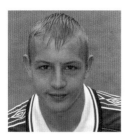

KIRK HILTON
Position: defender
Birthdate: 2 April 1981
Birthplace: Flixton
Signed trainee: 30 June 1997
Signed professional: 1 July 1999

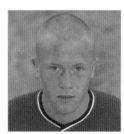

CHRIS HUMPHREYS
Position: forward
Birthdate: 22 September 1983
Birthplace: Manchester
Signed trainee: 3 July 2000
Signed professional: 1 July 2001

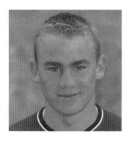

EDDIE JOHNSON
Position: forward
Birthdate: 20 September 1984
Birthplace: Chester
Signed trainee: 2 July 2001
Signed professional: 20 September 2001

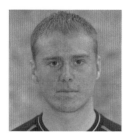

JAMES JOWSEY
Position: goalkeeper
Birthdate: 24 November 1983
Birthplace: Scarborough
Signed trainee: 3 July 2000
Signed professional: 24 November 2000

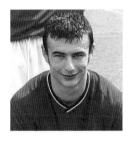

MARK LYNCH
Position: defender
Birthdate: 2 September 1981
Birthplace: Manchester
Signed trainee: 6 July 1998
Signed professional: 31 August 1999

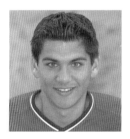

KALAM MOONIARUCK
Position: forward
Birthdate: 22 November 1983
Birthplace: Yeovil
Signed trainee: 3 July 2000
Signed professional: 22 November 2000

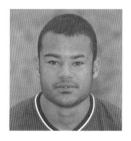

BEN MUIRHEAD
Position: forward
Birthdate: 5 January 1983
Birthplace: Doncaster
Signed trainee: 5 July 1999
Signed professional: 5 January 2000

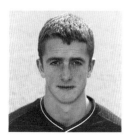

DANNY PUGH
Position: midfield
Birthdate: 19 October 1982
Birthplace: Manchester
Signed trainee: 5 July 1999
Signed professional: 12 July 2000

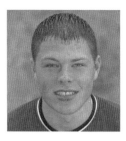

JOHN RANKIN
Position: midfield
Birthdate: 27 June 1983
Birthplace: Bellshill
Signed trainee: 5 July 1999
Signed professional: 27 June 2000

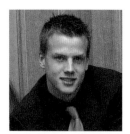

LUKE STEELE
Position: goalkeeper
Birthdate: 24 September 1984
Birthplace: Peterborough
Transferred: from Peterborough United 13 May 2002

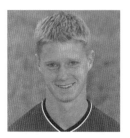

ALAN TATE
Position: defender
Birthdate: 2 September 1982
Birthplace: Easington
Signed trainee: 5 July 1999
Signed professional: 12 July 2000

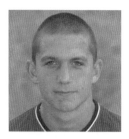

KRIS TAYLOR
Position: midfield
Birthdate: 12 January 1984
Birthplace: Stafford
Signed trainee: 3 July 2000
Signed professional: 26 January 2001

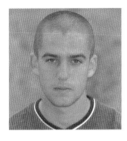

PAUL TIERNEY
Position: midfield
Birthdate: 15 September 1982
Birthplace: Salford
Signed trainee: 5 July 1999
Signed professional: 12 July 2000

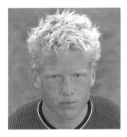

MADS TIMM
Position: forward
Birthdate: 31 October 1984
Birthplace: Odense, Denmark
Signed trainee: 2 July 2001
Signed professional: 12 December 2001

BEN WILLIAMS
Position: goalkeeper
Birthdate: 27 August 1982
Birthplace: Manchester
Signed trainee: 27 August 1999
Signed professional: to follow

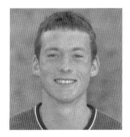

MATTHEW WILLIAMS
Position: forward
Birthdate: 5 November 1982
Birthplace: St Asaph
Signed trainee: 5 July 1999
Signed professional: 26 January 2000

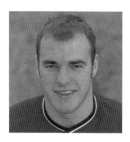

NEIL WOOD

Position: forward
Birthdate: 4 January 1983
Birthplace: Manchester
Signed trainee: 5 July 1999
Signed professional: 4 January 2000

TRAINEE PROFESSIONALS 2002-03

SECOND YEAR

Name	Position	Birthdate	Birthplace	Date Signed
Phillip BARDSLEY	defender	28 June 1985	Salford	2 July 2001
Danny BYRNE	midfield	30 November 1984	Frimley	2 July 2001
Ben COLLETT	midfield	11 September 1984	Bury	2 July 2001
David JONES	midfield	4 November 1984	Southport	2 July 2001
Lee LAWRENCE	defender	1 December 1984	Boston	2 July 2001
David POOLE	forward	12 November 1984	Manchester	2 July 2001
Kieran RICHARDSON	midfield	21 October 1984	Greenwich	2 July 2001
Lee SIMS	defender	6 September 1984	Manchester	2 July 2001

FIRST YEAR

Sylvan BLAKE	forward	29 March 1986	Cambridge	8 July 2002
Ramon CALLISTE	forward	16 December 1985	Cardiff	8 July 2002
Christopher EAGLES	midfield	19 November 1985	Hemel Hempstead	8 July 2002
Adam ECKERSLEY	defender	7 September 1985	Salford	8 July 2002
Callum FLANAGAN	forward	19 September 1985	Manchester	8 July 2002
Tom HEATON	goalkeeper	15 April 1986	Chester	8 July 2002
Mark HOWARD	defender	29 January 1986	Salford	8 July 2002
Tommy LEE	goalkeeper	3 January 1986	Keighley	8 July 2002
Paul McSHANE	defender	6 January 1986	Wicklow	8 July 2002
Adrian NEVINS	midfield	31 January 1986	Manchester	8 July 2002
Phil PICKEN	defender	12 November 1985	Manchester	8 July 2002
Graeme PORT	midfield	13 April 1986	York	8 July 2002

ACADEMY SCHOOLBOYS

Mark FOX	forward	8 November 1985	Stafford	
Steven HOGG	forward	1 October 1985	Bury	

DEPARTURES 2001-02

Name	Details	Date
Nick BAXTER	free transfer	30 June 2002
Laurent BLANC	free transfer	30 June 2002
Michael CLEGG	to Oldham Athletic	19 February 2002
Steven CLEGG	free transfer	30 June 2002
Craig COATES	Contract cancelled by mutual consent	19 July 2001
Andy COLE	to Blackburn Rovers	29 December 2001
Jonathan GREENING	to Middlesbrough	9 August 2001
Denis IRWIN	free transfer	30 June 2002
Ronny JOHNSEN	free transfer	30 June 2002
Jemal JOHNSON	Signed trainee forms for Blackburn Rovers	Summer 2001
Alan McDERMOTT	free transfer	30 June 2002
David MORAN	free transfer	30 June 2002
Paul RACHUBKA	to Charlton Athletic	20 May 2002
Gary SAMPSON	free transfer	30 June 2002
Jaap STAM	to SS Lazio	28 August 2001
Andrew TAYLOR	free transfer	30 June 2002
Raimond VAN DER GOUW	free transfer	30 June 2002
Ronnie WALLWORK	free transfer	30 June 2002
Marc WHITEMAN	Contract cancelled by mutual consent	27 June 2001
Mark WILSON	to Middlesbrough	9 August 2001

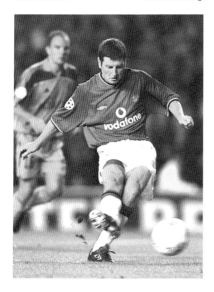

Denis Irwin

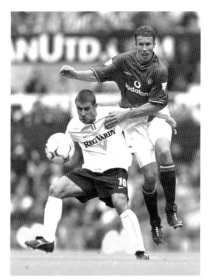

Ronny Johnsen

FA PREMIER RESERVE LEAGUE – NORTH

Brian McClair's inaugural season in charge of United's reserve team ended in triumph with the FA Premier Reserve League (North) being won for the first time. But it wasn't all plain sailing with the title looking to have slipped from their grasp as the season entered its final few weeks. McClair's lads started in great style and remained unbeaten until late December when Bolton Wanderers claimed all three points following a 4-2 win at Gigg Lane. Up to that stage it appeared that they could do little wrong with victories and goals in plentiful supply.

By mid-February they had played themselves into a very strong position – one point adrift of leaders Middlesbrough, but with four games in hand – and appearing all set to capture the club's first reserve championship since Jimmy Ryan's team collected the Pontin's Premier League crown in 1997. However, following a run of three defeats in four outings, it appeared that the outcome of this particular title race wasn't quite so inevitable as expected. Newcastle United had joined the race by this time and having already beaten United 5-2 on Tyneside in early March they improved their chances further when they added another point to their total

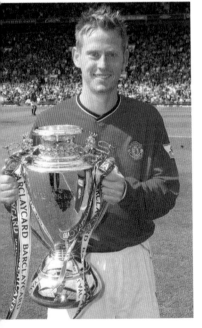

after holding United to a goalless draw at Gigg Lane.

The last few fixtures saw the race reduced to a head-to-head between United and the Magpies with Leeds United playing more than a bit part in the destination of the title. United's last two fixtures were home and away against Leeds with the Elland Road club's home meeting with Newcastle sandwiched in-between. United helped themselves with a 2-0 win at Leeds, which meant that defeat for the Magpies on the same ground a week later would hand the title to McClair's side.

And that was just what transpired, Leeds defeated Newcastle 1-0 and United were crowned Champions without kicking a ball. Skipper Michael Stewart collected the trophy, and the players received their medals, before the final Premiership match of the season against Charlton Athletic. It was the club's only silverware of the season.

Michael Stewart collects the FA Premier Reserve League (North) trophy before the Charlton game at Old Trafford in May 2002

names in bold indicate goalscorers

v MIDDLESBROUGH (away) • Drawn: 2-2 — Wednesday 29 August 2001

Culkin • Roche • Tierney • Wallwork • May • Yorke • **Lynch** • Stewart • Webber • Davis • **Fortune**
Substitutes: Tate • Williams B. • Sampson • Nardiello (Tierney) • Muirhead

v SUNDERLAND (home, at Gigg Lane, Bury) • Won: 3-0 — Thursday 6 September 2001

van der Gouw • Clegg M. • Tierney • O'Shea • May • Wallwork • Stewart • Butt • Webber • **Yorke 3** • Fortune
Substitutes: Lynch (Fortune) • Culkin • Roche • Nardiello (Yorke) • Davis (Butt)

v LIVERPOOL (home, at Gigg Lane, Bury) • Won: 3-2 — Thursday 13 September 2001

Carroll • Clegg M. • Irwin • O'Shea • May • **Wallwork** • Chadwick • Butt • **Solskjaer** • **Stewart** • Fortune
Substitutes: Roche (O'Shea) • Culkin • Webber • Davis • Djordjic (Butt)

v BRADFORD CITY (away) • Won: 7-2 — Thursday 18 October 2001

van der Gouw • Lynch • Neville P. • **O'Shea** • **May (pen)** • Wallwork • **Timm** • **Stewart** • **Fortune 2** • Yorke • Blomqvist
*Substitutes: **Webber (pen)** (Neville P.) • Williams B. • Djordjic (May) • Davis (Yorke) • Tate*

v ASTON VILLA (home, at Gigg Lane, Bury) • Won: 1-0 — Thursday 25 October 2001

Carroll • Roche • Clegg M. • O'Shea • May • Wallwork • Chadwick • Neville P. • **Webber** • Fortune • Djordjic
Substitutes: Davis (Chadwick) • Williams B. • Nardiello (Webber) • Tate • Fox (Neville P.)

v SHEFFIELD WEDNESDAY (home, at Gigg Lane, Bury) • Won: 5-1 — Thursday 1 November 2001

van der Gouw • Roche • Tierney • Clegg M. • Tate • Wallwork • Chadwick • Stewart • **Webber 2** • **Davis 2** • Djordjic
(Rand o.g.)
Substitutes: Nardiello (Stewart) • Williams B. • Fox (Wallwork) • Timm (Chadwick) • Taylor K

v EVERTON (away, at Auto Quest Stadium, Widnes) • Won: 3-1 — Tuesday 13 November 2001

Rachubka • Roche • Tierney • Clegg M. • Tate • Wallwork • Davis • Fletcher • Webber • **Nardiello** • **Djordjic**
*Substitutes: **Wood** (Fletcher) • Williams B. • Richardson (Wallwork) • Heath • Muirhead (Davis)*

v MANCHESTER CITY (home, at Gigg Lane, Bury) • Drawn: 1-1 — Thursday 22 November 2001

Carroll • Roche • Tierney • O'Shea • Clegg M. • Yorke • Chadwick • Stewart • **Webber** • Solskjaer • Djordjic
Substitutes: Davis • Williams B. • Nardiello (Solskjaer) • Tate • Sampson (Yorke)

RESERVES

Thursday 6 December 2001 **v BLACKBURN ROVERS (away, at Christie Park, Morecambe) • Won: 3-1**

Carroll • Roche • Tierney • Tate • Clegg M. • Wallwork • **Muirhead** • Stewart • **Nardiello** • **Davis** • Fortune
Substitutes: Rankin • Williams B. • Pugh (Wallwork) • Sampson • Williams M. (Nardiello)

Thursday 20 December 2001 **v BOLTON WANDERERS (home, at Gigg Lane, Bury) • Lost: 2-4**

van der Gouw • Roche • Tierney • Clegg M. • Wallwork • Wood • **Chadwick 2** • Stewart • Cole • Yorke • Fortune
Substitutes: Tate (Roche) • Williams B. • Nardiello (Wallwork) • Pugh (Yorke) • Muirhead

Thursday 17 January 2002 **v MIDDLESBROUGH (home, at Gigg Lane, Bury) • Won: 1-0**

Carroll • Roche • Irwin • Clegg M. • Tierney • Wallwork • **Davis** • Pugh • Webber • Nardiello • Djordjic
Substitutes: Clegg S. • Williams B. • Muirhead • Rankin (Irwin) • Williams M.

Monday 21 January 2002 **v SUNDERLAND (away) • Drawn: 0-0**

Williams B. • Roche • Pugh • Clegg M. • Tierney • Rankin • Davis • Stewart • Webber • Nardiello • Djordjic
Substitutes: Muirhead (Nardiello) • Moran • Williams M. (Webber) • Sampson • McDermott (Tierney)

Wednesday 13 February 2002 **v BOLTON WANDERERS (away) • Won: 3-0**

Williams B. • Roche • Irwin • O'Shea • Johnsen • **Wallwork** • **Davis** • Stewart • **Forlan** • Yorke • Fortune
Substitutes: Webber (Forlan) • Jowsey • Clegg M. • Tierney • Nardiello (Irwin)

Thursday 21 February 2002 **v ASTON VILLA (away) • Lost: 0-1**

van der Gouw • Roche • Pugh • Wallwork • Tierney • Fortune • Davis • Stewart • Webber • Nardiello • Djordjic
Substitutes: McDermott (Wallwork) • Williams B. • Rankin • Muirhead • Williams M. (Nardiello)

Thursday 28 February 2002 **v BRADFORD CITY (home, at Gigg Lane, Bury) • Drawn: 1-1**

Carroll • Roche • Pugh • O'Shea • Tierney • Fortune • Davis • Stewart • **Forlan** • Yorke • Djordjic
Substitutes: Webber (Forlan) • Williams B. • Williams M. (Fortune) • Rankin • McDermott (Roche)

Monday 4 March 2002 **v NEWCASTLE UNITED (away, at Kingston Park, Kenton) • Lost: 2-5**

Rachubka • Rankin • Pugh • O'Shea • Tierney • **Fortune** • Davis • Stewart • **Webber** • Yorke • Djordjic
Substitutes: McDermott • Williams B. • Williams M. (Davis) • Fox (Fortune) • Muirhead (Yorke)

names in bold indicate goalscorers

v BLACKBURN ROVERS (home, at Gigg Lane, Bury) • Lost: 1-2 — Thursday 14 March 2002

Steele • Neville P. • **Pugh** • O'Shea • Tierney • Stewart • Muirhead • Butt • Nardiello • Fortune • Djordjic
Substitutes: Rankin • Williams B. • Williams M. (Muirhead) • Sampson (Butt) • Fox (Fortune)

v LIVERPOOL (away, at Haig Avenue, Southport) • Drawn: 1-1 — Wednesday 20 March 2002

Carroll • Irwin • Pugh • O'Shea • Brown • Fortune • Davis • Stewart • **Webber** • Nardiello • Djordjic
Substitutes: Rankin • Williams B. • Muirhead (Davis) • Fox • Tierney (Brown)

v SHEFFIELD WEDNESDAY (away) • Won: 2-0 — Tuesday 26 March 2002

Rachubka • Brown • **Pugh** • Tierney • **May** • Fox • Davis • Stewart • Webber • Nardiello • Richardson
Substitutes: Rankin (Richardson) • Williams B. • Sims (Tierney) • Williams M. • Muirhead (Davis)

v NEWCASTLE UNITED (home, at Gigg Lane, Bury) • Drawn: 0-0 — Thursday 4 April 2002

Carroll • Brown • Pugh • Tierney • May • Wallwork • Davis • Stewart • Williams M. • Nardiello • Djordjic
Substitutes: Roche (Brown) • Williams B. • Tate (Williams M.) • Wood • Rankin

v MANCHESTER CITY (away, at Ewen Fields, Hyde) • Drawn: 1-1 — Tuesday 9 April 2002

van der Gouw • Roche • Pugh • Tierney • May • Wallwork • Wood • **Richardson** • Williams M. • Nardiello • Djordjic
Substitutes: Rankin • Williams B. • Tate (Williams M.) • Muirhead • Fox (Wood)

v EVERTON (home) • Won: 2-1 — Thursday 18 April 2002

Williams B. • Roche • Rankin • Tierney • May • **Wallwork** • Chadwick • Djordjic • Nardiello • **Davis** • Richardson
Substitutes: Tate • Moran • Williams M. (Nardiello) • Wood (Richardson) • Muirhead

v LEEDS UNITED (away) • Won: 2-0 — Thursday 25 April 2002

van Der Gouw • Roche • Rankin • Tierney • May • Wallwork • **Chadwick** • Djordjic • **Webber** • Davis • Richardson
Substitutes: Tate • Williams B. • Wood (Chadwick) • Williams M. (Richardson) • Muirhead (Webber)

v LEEDS UNITED (home, at Moss Lane, Altrincham) • Lost: 1-2 — Monday 6 May 2002

Rachubka • Clegg S. • Rankin • Roche • May • Wallwork • Lynch • Stewart • **Muirhead** • Nardiello • Djordjic
Substitutes: Williams M. • Williams B. • Tate (Clegg S.) • Wood • Fox (Lynch)

APPEARANCES

GOALSCORERS

Name	Appearances (as sub)	Name	Appearances (as sub)	Name	Goals
TIERNEY • Paul	18 (1)	BROWN • Wesley	3	WEBBER • Danny	8
STEWART • Michael	18	BUTT • Nicky	3	DAVIS • Jimmy	6
WALLWORK • Ronnie	17	NEVILLE • Phil	3	FORTUNE • Quinton	4
DJORDJIC • Bojan	16 (2)	WILLIAMS • Ben	3	CHADWICK • Luke	3
ROCHE • Lee	16 (2)	WILLIAMS • Matthew	2 (8)	WALLWORK • Ronnie	3
DAVIS • Jimmy	15 (3)	WOOD • Neil	2 (3)	YORKE • Dwight	3
WEBBER • Danny	13 (3)	FORLAN • Diego	2	FORLAN • Diego	2
FORTUNE • Quinton	13	SOLSKJAER • Ole Gunnar	2	MAY • David	2
NARDIELLO • Daniel	12 (7)	FOX • David	1 (6)	MUIRHEAD • Ben	2
MAY • David	11	TIMM • Mads	1 (1)	NARDIELLO • Daniel	2
PUGH • Danny	10 (2)	BLOMQVIST • Jesper	1	PUGH • Danny	2
CLEGG • Michael	10	COLE • Andy	1	STEWART • Michael	2
O'SHEA • John	10	CLEGG • Steven	1	DJORDJIC • Bojan	1
CARROLL • Roy	8	CULKIN • Nick	1	LYNCH • Mark	1
YORKE • Dwight	8	FLETCHER • Darren	1	O'SHEA • John	1
CHADWICK • Luke	7	JOHNSEN • Ronny	1	RICHARDSON • Kieran	1
VAN DER GOUW • Raimond	7	STEELE • Luke	1	SOLSKJAER • Ole Gunnar	1
RANKIN • John	5 (2)	McDERMOTT • Alan	0 (3)	TIMM • Mads	1
RICHARDSON • Kieran	4 (1)	SAMPSON • Gary	0 (2)	WOOD • Neil	1
IRWIN • Denis	4	SIMS • Lee	0 (1)		
RACHUBKA • Paul	4			**Own Goal**	
MUIRHEAD • Ben	3 (6)			RAND • Craig	1
TATE • Alan	3 (4)			(Sheffield Wednesday)	
LYNCH • Mark	3 (1)				

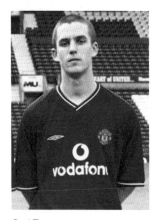

Paul Tierney

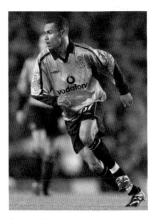

Danny Webber

FA BARCLAYCARD PREMIERSHIP RESERVE LEAGUE – NORTH

FINAL TABLE 2001-02		P	W	D	L	F	A	Pts
	MANCHESTER UNITED	24	12	7	5	47	28	43
	Newcastle United	24	13	3	7	46	27	42
	Middlesbrough	24	12	6	6	36	26	42
	Sunderland	24	12	4	8	43	28	40
	Bolton Wanderers	24	12	3	9	45	40	39
	Manchester City	24	10	7	7	40	28	37
	Blackburn Rovers	24	11	4	9	41	30	37
	Leeds United	24	10	4	10	25	33	34
	Liverpool	24	9	6	9	54	49	33
	Everton	24	8	8	8	30	30	32
	Aston Villa	24	7	4	13	26	59	25
	Bradford City	24	5	6	13	27	56	21
	Sheffield Wednesday	24	2	4	18	26	59	10

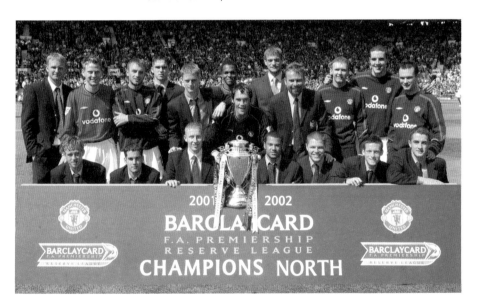

FA Barclaycard Premiership Reserve League (North) Champions. Back row, left to right: David May, Michael Stewart, Ronnie Wallwork, Bojan Djordjic, Alan Tate, Quinton Fortune, Raimond van der Gouw, Roy Carroll, Brian McClair (manager), Alec Wylie (kit manager), John O'Shea, Neil Hough (physiotherapist). Front row: David Fox, Daniel Nardiello, Lee Roche, Ben Muirhead, John Rankin, Matthew Williams, Danny Pugh

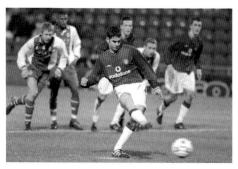

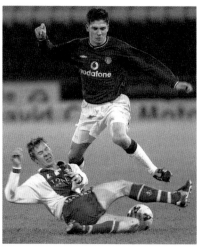

(Above and right) The Reserves in action away at Oldham Athletic in the Manchester Senior Cup. Oldham won 2-1

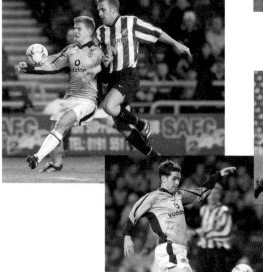

(Above left, above and left) The Reserves in league action away at Sunderland in January 2002. The match ended in a 0-0 draw

names in bold indicate goalscorers

MANCHESTER SENIOR CUP

v MANCHESTER CITY (away, at Ewen Fields, Hyde) • Lost: 0-5 Wednesday 3 September 2001

Williams B. • Clegg M. • Roche • McDermott • Tate • Wallwork • Lynch • Sampson • Davis • Nardiello • Blomqvist
Substitutes: Tierney (Roche) • Moran • Taylor K. • Heath (McDermott) • Richardson (Blomqvist)

v OLDHAM ATHLETIC (home, at Moss Lane, Altrincham) • Won: 4-1 Thursday 24 January 2002

Williams B. • Roche • Clegg • O'Shea • Brown • Wallwork • Chadwick • **Stewart** • **Webber** • **Davis** • **Djordjic**
Substitutes: McDermott (O'Shea) • Baxter • Pugh • Nardiello • Rankin

v MANCHESTER CITY (home, at Moss Lane, Altrincham) • Drawn: 1-1* Thursday 31 January 2002

Carroll • Brown • Irwin • O'Shea • Clegg M. • Wallwork • Davis • Stewart • **Webber** • Forlan • Djordjic
Substitutes: McDermott • Williams B. • Nardiello (Forlan) • Roche (O'Shea)
* Lost 3-4 on penalties. Penalty-scorers: Djordjic • Irwin • Davis

v BURY (home, at Moss Lane, Altrincham) • Drawn: 1-1* Thursday 7 March 2002

Carroll • Rankin • Pugh • O'Shea • Tierney • Yorke • Muirhead • Stewart • Webber • Davis • Djordjic
(Thompson o.g.)
Substitutes: McDermott • Williams B. • Williams M. • Nardiello (Muirhead) • Fox
* Lost 2-3 on penalties. Penalty-scorers: Nardiello • Davis

v OLDHAM ATHLETIC (away) • Lost: 1-2 Monday 11 March 2002

Steele • Rankin • Pugh • McDermott • Tierney • Fox • Muirhead • Stewart • **Nardiello (pen)** • Williams M. • Djordjic
Substitutes: Taylor K. • Williams B. • Cogger (McDermott) • Sampson • Heath (Williams M.)

v BURY (away) • Won: 1-0 Monday 15 April 2002

Williams M. • Clegg S. • Rankin • Tate • Cogger • Sampson • Mooniaruck • Humphreys • Heath • **Muirhead** • Richardson
Substitutes: Taylor K. • Jowsey • Poole (Heath) • Sims • Johnson (Mooniaruck)

	P	W	D	L	F	A	Pts
Manchester City	6	6	0	0	18	5	18
Oldham Athletic	6	3	0	3	11	10	9
MANCHESTER UNITED	6	2	0	4	8	10	6
Bury	6	1	0	5	2	14	3

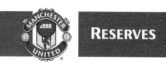

FRIENDLIES

v DONCASTER ROVERS (away) • Drawn: 2-2

Culkin • Roche • Clegg M. • O'Shea • May • **Wallwork** • Lynch • Stewart • Webber • **Nardiello** • Djordjic
Substitutes: Tate • Muirhead • Tierney

v SHEFFIELD FC (away) • Won: 3-2

Carroll • Roche • Clegg M. • O'Shea • May • **Wallwork 2** • Lynch • Stewart • **Webber** • Nardiello • Djordjic
Substitutes: Tate • Rachubka • Tierney • Sampson • Muirhead (Nardiello) • Williams M. (Roche) • Rankin

v HEREFORD UNITED (away) • Won: 6-0

van der Gouw • Irwin • Neville P. • Brown • Johnsen • Keane • **Fortune 2** • **Butt** • **Cole 2** • **Yorke** • Djordjic
Substitutes: Roche • Culkin • Sampson • Lynch • Stewart (Djordjic) • Clegg M. • Tierney • Webber • Tate (Johnsen)

HILVERSUM TOURNAMENT 2001

v VITESSE ARNHEM (Holland) Semi-Final • Drawn: 1-1*

Culkin • Roche • Clegg M. • O'Shea • May • Wallwork • Lynch • Sampson • Davis • **Nardiello** • Djordjic
Substitutes: Tate • Jowsey • Tierney • Muirhead (Lynch) • Rankin
* Won 4-3 on penalties. *Penalty-scorers:* O'Shea • Nardiello • Davis • May

v AJAX (Holland) Final • Lost: 0-3

Culkin • Roche • Clegg M. • O'Shea • May • Wallwork • Lynch • Sampson • Davis • Nardiello • Djordjic
Substitutes: Tate (May) • Jowsey • Tierney (O'Shea) • Muirhead (Lynch) • Rankin (Djordjic)

v LINFIELD (away) • Won: 2-1

Culkin • Roche • Tierney • O'Shea • May • **Wallwork** • Lynch • Sampson • Davis • **Webber** • Djordjic
Substitutes: Tate (May) • Williams B. • Fox • Rankin (Djordjic) • Nardiello (O'Shea) • Muirhead

v NEWCASTLE TOWN (away) • Won: 9-0

Culkin • Clegg M. • Roche • O'Shea • McDermott • **Fox** • **Lynch** • Sampson • **Webber 3** • **Davis 3** • Rankin
*Substitutes: Tierney (McDermott) • Williams B. (Culkin) • Fletcher (Fox) • **Mooniaruck** (Lynch) • Heath (Rankin)*

names in bold indicate goalscorers

v NEWRY TOWN (away) • Won: 5-0 — Tuesday 9 October 2001

Williams B. • Clegg M. • Tierney • O'Shea • McDermott • **Wallwork** • Lynch • **Nardiello** • **Davis** • Djordjic • **Blomqvist 2**
Substitutes: Tate (O'Shea) • Moran • Muirhead (Lynch) • Fox (McDermott) • Heath (Davis)

v BARNSLEY Eric Winstanley Testimonial (away) • Lost: 0-1 — Monday 12 November 2001

Carroll • Neville P. • Irwin • Stewart • O'Shea • Blanc • Davis • Fortune • Yorke • Solskjaer • Giggs
Substitutes: Wallwork (Fortune) • Rachubka (Carroll) • Clegg M. (Blanc) • Roche (Davis) • Djordjic (Giggs) •
Webber (Solskjaer) •Tierney (Irwin)

v BURNLEY Friendly/Training Match (home, at Trafford Training Centre) • Won: 2-1 — Wednesday 28 November 2001

van der Gouw • Roche • Tierney • O'Shea • Clegg • Wallwork • Chadwick • Stewart • **Cole** • **Yorke** • Djordjic
Substitutes: Davis • Nardiello • Wood • Sampson • Rankin • Tate

v NEWTOWN (away) • Lost: 3-4 — Tuesday 12 March 2002

Baxter • **Sims** • Lawrence • Bardsley • Cogger • Taylor K. • Poole • Sampson • **Heath** • **Johnson** • Richardson
Substitutes: Williams M. (Sampson) • Moran (Baxter) • Jones D. (Cogger) • Collett (Johnson)

v DRUMCHAPEL AMATEURS Friendly/Training Match (home, at Training Centre) • Won: 8-0 — Sunday 31 March 2002

Williams B. • Brown • Pugh • McLean (trialist) • May • **Wallwork** • **Williams M.** • Steart • **Davis 3** • **Nardiello 3** • Djordjic
Substitutes: Roche (Pugh) • Baxter (Williams B.) • Tierney (May) • Sampson (Williams M.)

v RHYL (away) • Lost: 1-2 — Monday 29 April 2002

Moran • Clegg S. • Taylor K. • Fox • **Tate** • Cogger • Mooniaruck • Sampson • Heath • Williams M. • Humphreys
Substitutes: Rankin (Mooniaruck) • Williams B. (Moran) • Tierney (Cogger) • Wood (Sampson)

FA PREMIER ACADEMY LEAGUE – UNDER 19s

The Under 19s, coached by David Williams, went within a hairs-breadth of glory after being among the Group C leaders all season. They reached the climax of the season with their destiny in their own hands. Requiring four points from their

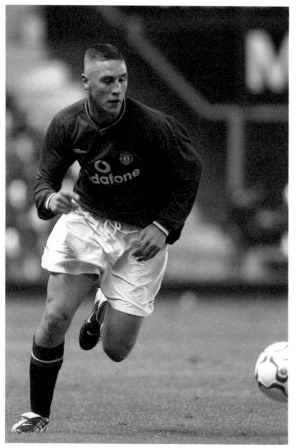

final two games to pip Liverpool to the group honours, they did themselves no favours when losing their penultimate game 3-1 at home to Derby County.

One point would have been sufficient to nose them ahead of Liverpool, but the defeat meant that they went into the final match, away at Middlesbrough, needing to do better than Liverpool who were also away at Leeds.

Williams' lads did their bit with a 2-1 win at Boro's picturesque Rockcliffe training complex, but in the end it wasn't enough with Liverpool also snapping up three points and the season's honours.

Defender John Cogger made 21 starts for the Under 19s – more than any other player in the squad

names in bold indicate goalscorers

v SOUTHAMPTON (home) • Won: 5-1 — Saturday 25 August 2001

Jowsey • Clegg • Taylor K. • Fox • **Tate** • Tierney • Muirhead • Sampson • **Nardiello** • **Heath 2** • Rankin
(Davies o.g.)
Substitutes: Taylor A. (Humphreys) • Baxter • Cogger (Taylor K.) • Humphreys (Nardiello)

v SUNDERLAND (home) • Won: 3-0 — Saturday 8 September 2001

Baxter • Cogger • Rankin • Fox • Tate • Taylor K. • Muirhead • Sampson • **Nardiello 2** • **Heath** • Richardson
Substitutes: Tierney • Jowsey • Kouman • Camilleri (trialist) • Eckersley

v SHEFFIELD UNITED (away) • Won: 2-1 — Saturday 15 September 2001

Jowsey • Cogger • Taylor K. • Fox • Tate • Tierney • Muirhead • Richardson • **Nardiello** • **Heath** • Rankin
Substitutes: Clegg • Moran (Taylor K.) • Fletcher (Richardson) • Camilleri (trialist)

v NOTTINGHAM FOREST (away) • Drawn: 1-1 — Saturday 29 September 2001

Moran • Clegg • Taylor K. • Fox • Tate • Tierney • Muirhead • Sampson • **Nardiello** • Heath • Rankin
Substitutes: Fletcher (Fox) • Baxter • Cogger • Mooniaruck (Muirhead)

v COVENTRY CITY (home) • Won: 3-1 — Saturday 6 October 2001

Baxter • Clegg • Taylor K. • **Fox** • Cogger • Tierney • **Mooniaruck** • Fletcher • Nardiello • **Heath** • Rankin
Substitutes: Tate • Jowsey • Sampson (Fletcher) • Pugh (Rankin) • Williams M. (Nardiello)

v EVERTON (home) • Won: 3-2 — Saturday 13 October 2001

Jowsey • Clegg • Taylor K. • Sampson • Tate • Cogger • **Mooniaruck** • Fletcher • Muirhead • Heath • Richardson
*Substitutes: Fox (Sampson) • Moran • **Pugh 2** (Fletcher) • Tierney (Cogger)*

v MANCHESTER CITY (away) • Drawn: 1-1 — Saturday 20 October 2001

Moran • Clegg • Taylor K. • Fox • Tate • Tierney • Mooniaruck • Fletcher • **Nardiello** • Muirhead • Rankin
Substitutes: Sampson (Fletcher) • Jowsey • Pugh (Rankin) • Cogger • Heath (Mooniaruck)

v SHEFFIELD WEDNESDAY (home) • Won: 2-0 — Tuesday 23 October 2001

Jowsey • Clegg • Taylor K. • **Fox** • Tate • Cogger • Muirhead • Sampson • Nardiello • **Heath** • Pugh
Substitutes: Fletcher (Pugh) • Moran • Wood (Fox) • Leather

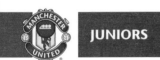

JUNIORS

v WREXHAM (home) • Won: 3-2

Moran • Clegg • Tierney • Sampson • Cogger • Taylor K. • Muirhead • Fletcher • **Heath** • Humphreys • **Pugh**
*Substitutes: Tate (Pugh) • Jowsey • **Nardiello** (Humphreys) • Wood (Cogger) • Fox*

v BLACKBURN ROVERS (away) • Won: 3-0

Jowsey • Clegg • Pugh • Fletcher • Cogger • Taylor K. • Muirhead • **Wood** • **Nardiello (pen)** • **Heath** • Rankin
Substitutes: Fox (Wood) • Moran • Sampson (Pugh) • Humphreys

v STOKE CITY (away) • Drawn: 0-0

Baxter • Sims • Lawrence • Sampson • Cogger • Taylor K. • Muirhead • Fletcher • Heath • Humphreys • Richardson
Substitutes: Tate • Moran • Pugh (Richardson) • Wood (Humphreys)

v BOLTON WANDERERS (home) • Won: 2-1

Moran • Clegg • Pugh • Fox • Tate • Cogger • Muirhead • **Humphreys 2** • Heath • Wood • Rankin
Substitutes: Sampson (Wood) • Jowsey • Tierney (Pugh) • Fletcher • Poole (Humphreys)

v LIVERPOOL (away) • Lost: 1-3

Jowsey • Clegg • Pugh • Fox • **Tate** • Cogger • Fletcher • Heath • Nardiello • Sampson • Rankin
Substitutes: Tierney (Rankin) • Moran • Williams M. (Heath)

v SHEFFIELD WEDNESDAY (away) • Won: 2-1

Moran • Clegg • Pugh • Sampson • Tate • Tierney • Mooniaruck • Williams M. • **Nardiello (pen)** • Wood • Rankin
*Substitutes: Heath • Baxter • **Fox** (Wood) • Humphreys (Williams M.) • Kouman (Mooniaruck)*

v CREWE ALEXANDRA (home) • Lost: 0-1

Baxter • Clegg • Pugh • Fox • Cogger • Sims • Mooniaruck • Williams M. • Heath • Fletcher • Rankin
Substitutes: Sampson • Lee • Richardson (Rankin) • Humphreys (Williams M.) • Timm (Mooniaruck)

v WREXHAM (away) • Won: 3-2

Baxter • Clegg • Pugh • Fox • Cogger • Sims • Mooniaruck • Fletcher • **Williams M. 2** • **Humphreys** • Rankin
Substitutes: Heath (Humphreys) • Moran • Muirhead (Mooniaruck) • Bardsley

names in bold indicate goalscorers

v BLACKBURN ROVERS (home) • Won: 4-1 — Saturday 12 January 2002

Jowsey • Clegg • Pugh • Fox • Cogger • Sims • Mooniaruck • **Fletcher** • **Heath** • **Humphreys** • Richardson
(Martin o.g.)
Substitutes: Taylor K. (Cogger) • Moran • Muirhead • Rankin • Sampson

v STOKE CITY (home) • Won: 2-1 — Saturday 19 January 2002

Moran • Clegg • Pugh • Sampson • **Cogger** • Taylor K. • Muirhead • Jones D. • **Williams M.** • Poole • Rankin
Substitutes: Fox (Pugh) • Baxter • Humphreys (Muirhead) • Tierney (Taylor K.)

v LIVERPOOL (home) • Won: 3-0 — Saturday 2 February 2002

Baxter • Clegg • Pugh • Sampson • Cogger • Taylor K. • **Muirhead** • Fletcher • **Nardiello 2** • Williams M. • Richardson
Substitutes: Fox (Fletcher) • Jowsey • Heath (Richardson) • Mooniaruck • Johnson (Nardiello)

v CREWE ALEXANDRA (away) • Won: 4-1 — Saturday 9 February 2002

Moran • Sims • Pugh • Sampson • Bardsley • Tierney • Muirhead • **Humphreys** • **Nardiello 3** • Heath • Rankin
Substitutes: Fox (Humphreys) • Baxter • Mooniaruck (Nardiello) • Richardson (Rankin)

v COVENTRY CITY (away) • Drawn: 1-1 — Saturday 16 February 2002

Moran • Cogger • Pugh • Humphreys • Taylor K. • Tierney • Mooniaruck • Muirhead • **Nardiello** • Richardson • Rankin
Substitutes: Heath • Jowsey • Fox (Humphreys) • Sims

v MANCHESTER CITY (home) • Won: 4-2 — Wednesday 20 February 2002

Jowsey • Sims • Taylor K. • Fox • Cogger • Bardsley • Byrne • **Humphreys 2** • **Heath 2** • Fletcher • Richardson
Substitutes: Jones D. (Sims) • Moran • Mooniaruck (Richardson) • Muirhead

v EVERTON (away) • Lost: 0-3 — Saturday 23 February 2002

Moran • Cogger • Pugh • Fox • Taylor K. • Tierney • Mooniaruck • Muirhead • Williams M. • Fletcher • Rankin
Substitutes: Humphreys • Jowsey • Heath (Mooniaruck) • Bardsley (Pugh)

v HUDDERSFIELD TOWN (away) • Lost: 0-2 — Saturday 9 March 2002

Jowsey • Cogger • Lawrence • Fox • Bardsley • Taylor K. • Mooniaruck • Sampson • Nardiello • Williams M. • Richardson
Substitutes: Heath (Nardiello) • Baxter • Rankin (Bardsley) • Muirhead (Mooniaruck)

JUNIORS

Saturday 16 March 2002 v **BARNSLEY (home) • Won: 3-1**

Baxter • Rankin • Lawrence • Fox • Bardsley • **Taylor K.** • **Mooniaruck** • Sampson • **Heath** • Johnson • Richardson
Substitutes: Humphreys • Moran • Jones D.

Saturday 23 March 2002 v **BOLTON WANDERERS (away) • Won: 4-3**

Jowsey • **Cogger** • Rankin • Sampson • Bardsley • Taylor K. • Mooniaruck • Humphreys • **Heath** • **Williams M. 2** • Richardson
Substitutes: Fox (Sampson) • Baxter • Tierney • Muirhead (Mooniaruck) • Johnson (Heath)

Saturday 6 April 2002 v **DERBY COUNTY (home) • Lost: 1-3**

Jowsey • Clegg • Lawrence • Sampson • Tate • Cogger • Mooniaruck • **Humphreys** • Heath • Wood • Richardson
Substitutes: Fox • Baxter (Jowsey) • Muirhead • Taylor K. • Johnson

Saturday 13 April 2002 v **MIDDLESBROUGH (away) • Won: 2-1**

Jowsey • Sims • Taylor K. • Fox • Tate • Bardsley • **Poole** • Johnson • **Heath (pen)** • Wood • Rankin
Substitutes: Humphreys (Heath) • Moran • Richardson (Wood) • Collett • Lawrence

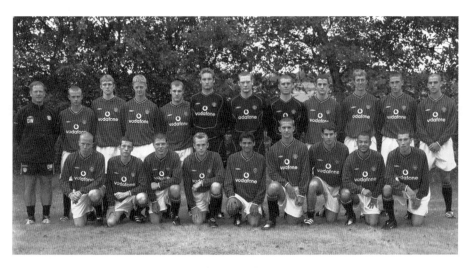

Manchester United Academy 2001-02 Under 19s squad. Back row, left to right: David Williams (coach), David Fox, Darren Fletcher, Alan Tate, Neil Wood, Nick Baxter, David Moran, James Jowsey, Danny Pugh, Colin Heath, John Cogger, Paul Tierney. Front row: Chris Humphreys, Matthew Williams, John Rankin, Andy Taylor, Kalam Mooniaruck, Kris Taylor, Daniel Nardiello, Ben Muirhead, Gary Sampson

UNDER 19s APPEARANCES

GOALSCORERS

Name	Appearances (as sub)	Name	Appearances (as sub)
COGGER • John	21 (1)	WILLIAMS • Matthew	8 (2)
HEATH • Colin	20 (5)	BAXTER • Nick	7 (1)
TAYLOR • Kris	20 (1)	SIMS • Lee	7
RANKIN • John	19 (1)	BARDSLEY • Phil	6 (1)
FOX • David	17 (8)	WOOD • Neil	5 (3)
CLEGG • Steven	17	LAWRENCE • Lee	4
SAMPSON • Gary	16 (4)	JOHNSON • Eddie	2 (2)
MUIRHEAD • Ben	16 (3)	POOLE • David	2 (1)
PUGH • Danny	14 (4)	JONES • David	1 (1)
NARDIELLO • Daniel	14 (1)	BYRNE • Danny	1
FLETCHER • Darren	13 (3)	KOUMAN • Amadou	0 (1)
MOONIARUCK • Kalam	13 (3)	TAYLOR • Andy	0 (1)
RICHARDSON • Kieran	12 (3)	TIMM • Mads	0 (1)
TATE • Alan	12 (1)		
JOWSEY • James	12		
HUMPHREYS • Chris	10 (5)		
TIERNEY • Paul	10 (4)		
MORAN • David	9 (1)		

Name	Goals
NARDIELLO • Daniel	15
HEATH • Colin	14
HUMPHREYS • Chris	8
WILLIAMS • Matthew	5
FOX • David	3
MOONIARUCK • Kalam	3
PUGH • Danny	3
COGGER • John	2
TATE • Alan	2
FLETCHER • Darren	1
MUIRHEAD • Ben	1
POOLE • David	1
TAYLOR • Kris	1
WOOD • Neil	1

Own Goals

DAVIES • Arron (Southampton)	1
MARTIN • Anthony (Blackburn Rovers)	1

FA PREMIER ACADEMY LEAGUE UNDER 19s

GROUP C FINAL TABLE 2001-02

	P	W	D	L	F	A	Pts
Liverpool	28	18	7	3	74	37	61
MANCHESTER UNITED	**28**	**19**	**4**	**5**	**62**	**36**	**61**
Manchester City	28	15	5	8	53	38	50
Crewe Alexandra	28	14	7	7	55	47	49
Coventry City	28	12	6	10	49	37	42
Everton	28	11	9	8	43	31	42
Blackburn Rovers	28	8	9	11	45	43	33
Stoke City	28	7	6	15	40	46	27
Bolton Wanderers	28	5	6	17	39	59	21
Wrexham	28	1	2	25	25	103	5

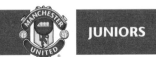

FA YOUTH CUP

Tuesday 4 December 2001   v QUEENS PARK RANGERS Third Round (away) • Won: 3-1

Jowsey • Sims • Lawrence • Fox • Cogger • Bardsley • **Timm** • Humphreys • **Heath 2** • Fletcher • Richardson
Substitutes: Mooniaruck (Timm) • Lee • Johnson (Humphreys) • Collett (Richardson) • Jones D.

Wednesday 23 January 2002   v BIRMINGHAM CITY Fourth Round (away) • Won: 3-2

Jowsey • Sims • Lawrence • Fox • Bardsley • Taylor K. • Mooniaruck • Fletcher • **Heath** • **Humphreys 2** • Richardson
Substitutes: Cogger • Lee • Johnson • Jones D. • Timm (Mooniaruck)

Wednesday 6 February 2002   v HARTLEPOOL UNITED Fifth Round (home) • Won: 3-2*

Jowsey • Sims • Lawrence • Fox • Bardsley • Taylor K. • Mooniaruck • Fletcher • **Heath** • Humphreys • **Richardson**
*Substitutes: Cogger (Sims) • Lee • Jones D. • Collett (Lawrence) • **Poole** (Humphreys)*
* After extra time

Friday 1 March 2002   v BARNSLEY Sixth Round (home) • Drawn: 3-3*

Jowsey • Sims • Lawrence • Fox • Bardsley • Taylor K. • Byrne • Fletcher • **Heath 2** • Humphreys • Richardson
*Substitutes: Cogger (Sims) • Lee • Mooniaruck (Byrne) • **Johnson** (Humphreys) • Poole*
* After extra time. Lost 1-3 on penalties. *Penalty-scorer: Fox*

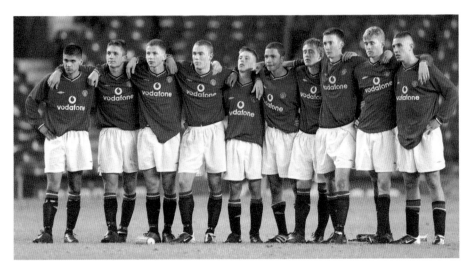

A tense moment as the Under 19s watch the FA Youth Cup Sixth Round penalty shootout, left to right: Kalam Mooniaruck, Kris Taylor, Phillip Bardsley, Eddie Johnson, Lee Lawrence, Kieran Richardson, David Fox, Colin Heath, Darren Fletcher, John Cogger

FIFA YOUTH CUP 2002 – FC BLUE STARS (ZURICH)

v ENERGIE COTTBUS (Germany) Group A • Drawn: 1-1 — Wednesday 8 May 2002

Williams B. • Cogger • Rankin • Taylor • Tate • Fox • Muirhead • Wood • **Williams M.** • Nardiello • Djordjic

Substitute: Heath (Nardiello)

v FC BLUE STARS (Switzerland) Group A • Lost: 0-1 — Wednesday 8 May 2002

Baxter • Clegg • Rankin • Taylor • Tate • Fox • Mooniaruck • Humphreys • Williams M. • Nardiello • Djordjic

Substitutes: Muirhead (Humphreys) • Heath (Nardiello)

v GRÊMIO PORTO ALEGRE (Brazil) Group A • Lost: 1-2 — Wednesday 8 May 2002

Jowsey • Clegg • Rankin • Taylor • Tate • Fox • Muirhead • Mooniaruck • Heath • **Sampson** • Djordjic

Substitute: Williams M. (Mooniaruck)

v KOREA Ninth/Twelfth Place Play-Off • Drawn: 2-2* — Thursday 9 May 2002

Williams B. • Clegg • Rankin • Taylor • Tate • Fox • Muirhead • Cogger • Heath • **Nardiello 2** • Djordjic

Substitutes: Mooniaruck (Muirhead) • Williams M. (Nardiello)

* Lost 6-7 on penalties. *Penalty-scorers:* Tate • Cogger • Muirhead • Fox • Djordjic • Rankin

v FC BLUE STARS (Switzerland) Eleventh/Twelfth Place Play-Off • Won: 2-0 — Thursday 9 May 2002

Jowsey • Clegg • Rankin • Taylor • Tate • Sampson • Mooniaruck • Humphreys • Williams M. • **Nardiello 2** • Wood

TOURNAMENT SQUAD

Nick BAXTER

Steven CLEGG

John COGGER

Bojan DJORDJIC

David FOX

Colin HEATH

Chris HUMPHREYS

James JOWSEY

Kalam MOONIARUCK

Ben MUIRHEAD

Daniel NARDIELLO

John RANKIN

Gary SAMPSON

Alan TATE

Kris TAYLOR

Ben WILLIAMS

Matthew WILLIAMS

Neil WOOD

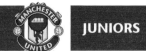

JUNIORS

NOKIA DEBITEL CUP 40TH
INTERNATIONAL YOUTH TOURNAMENT, DUSSELDORF

Saturday 30 March 2002   v JUVENTUS (Italy) Group Stage • Drawn: 1-1

Jowsey • Sims • Rankin • Fox • Clegg • Taylor • Muirhead • Humphreys • Heath • **Johnson** • Richardson
Substitute: Cogger (Clegg)

Saturday 30 March 2002   v BORUSSIA DORTMUND (Germany) Group Stage • Lost: 0-1

Moran • Sims • Rankin • Cogger • Taylor • Jones • Muirhead • Byrne • Heath • Poole • Richardson
Substitutes: Clegg (Sims) • Mooniaruck (Muirhead) • Johnson

Sunday 31 March 2002   v JAPAN Qualifying Round • Won: 4-1

Jowsey • Sims • Rankin • Fox • **Cogger** • Taylor • **Muirhead** • Humphreys • **Heath (pen)** • **Johnson** • Richardson
Substitutes: Poole (Johnson) • Lawrence (Rankin)

Sunday 31 March 2002   v FORTUNA DUSSELDORF (Germany) Quarter-Final • Drawn: 0-0*

Jowsey • Sims • Rankin • Fox • Cogger • Taylor • Muirhead • Humphreys • Heath • Johnson • Richardson
* Won 4-1 on penalties. Penalty-scorers: Fox • Richardson • Heath • Humphreys

Monday 1 April 2002   v BORUSSIA DORTMUND (Germany) Semi-Final • Drawn: 0-0*

Jowsey • Sims • Rankin • Fox • Cogger • Taylor • Muirhead • Humphreys • Heath • Johnson • Richardson
Substitutes: Jones (Humphreys) • Poole (Johnson)
* Lost: 6-7 on penalties.

Monday 1 April 2002   v BAYER 04 LEVERKUSEN (Germany) Third/Fourth Place Play-Off • Lost: 0-1

Moran • Sims • Lawrence • Clegg • Jones • Taylor • Mooniaruck • Byrne • Poole • Johnson • Rankin
Substitutes: Humphreys (Jones) • Heath (Poole) • Muirhead (Johnson)

TOURNAMENT SQUAD

Danny BYRNE	Eddie JOHNSON	Ben MUIRHEAD
Steven CLEGG	David JONES	David POOLE
John COGGER	James JOWSEY	John RANKIN
David FOX	Lee LAWRENCE	Kieran RICHARDSON
Colin HEATH	Kalam MOONIARUCK	Lee SIMS
Chris HUMPHREYS	David MORAN	Kris TAYLOR

FRIENDLIES

v CHADDERTON (away) • Won: 7-1
Monday 21 July 2001

Moran • Taylor A. • Taylor K. • Fox • Tate • Tierney • Muirhead • Sampson • **Gomez 3** • **Nardiello 3** • Rankin
Substitutes: Cogger (Tate) • Jowsey (Moran) • Humphreys (Sampson) • Mooniaruck (Muirhead) •
*Williams M. (Nardiello) • **Heath** (Rankin)*

v BOSTON UNITED (away) • Drawn: 1-1
Wednesday 26 July 2001

Moran • Taylor A. • Taylor K. • Fox • Tate • Tierney • **Muirhead** • Sampson • Nardiello • Williams M. • Rankin
Substitutes: Cogger (Taylor A.) • Jowsey • Mooniaruck (Muirhead) • Humphreys (Taylor K.) •
Heath (Williams M.) • Clegg S.

v WORKSOP TOWN (away) • Won: 3-0
Saturday 28 July 2001

Jowsey • Clegg S. • Tierney • Humphreys • Tate • Cogger • Mooniaruck • Sampson • **Heath** • **Williams M.** • **Rankin**
Substitutes: Taylor A. (Clegg S.) • Baxter (Jowsey) • Muirhead (Mooniaruck) • Taylor K. (Tierney)

v UPTON ATHLETIC ASSOCIATION (away) • Won: 7-1
Wednesday 1 August 2001

Baxter • Clegg S. • Taylor K. • Taylor A. • Cogger • **Tierney** • Mooniaruck • **Humphreys 2** • **Gomez 2** • **Heath** • Muirhead
*Substitutes: Rankin (Muirhead) • Moran • Sampson (Tierney) • **Williams M.** (Heath)*

v PORTSMOUTH (home) • Drawn: 0-0
Wednesday 8 August 2001

Moran • Clegg S. • Taylor K. • Taylor A. • Tate • Tierney • Muirhead • Sampson • Nardiello • Williams M. • Rankin
Substitutes: Humphreys (Taylor A.) • Baxter • Mooniaruck (Muirhead) • Cogger • Heath (Williams M.)

JERSEY TOURNAMENT

v SL BENFICA (Portugal) Group B • Lost: 0-1
Wednesday 15 August 2001

Baxter • Clegg S. • Taylor K. • Fox • Tate • Tierney • Muirhead • Sampson • Nardiello • Heath • Rankin
Substitutes: Humphreys (Heath) • Richardson (Rankin)

v CELTIC (Scotland) Group B • Lost: 2-3
Saturday 18 August 2001

Moran • Clegg S. • Rankin • Fox • Tate • Tierney • Muirhead • Humphreys • **Nardiello** • **Heath** • Richardson
Substitute: Sampson (Heath)

v MAJOR SOCCER LEAGUE Under-21 (United States of America) (home) • Won: 5-0
Tuesday 30 October 2001

Williams B. • Roche • Tierney • Clegg M. • McDermott • Fox • Davis • **Nardiello** • **Webber 2** • **Wood** • Blomqvist
Substitutes: Tate (McDermott) • Moran (Williams B.) • Pugh (Clegg M.) • Sampson (Blomqvist)
*Clegg S. (Roche) • **Heath** (Davis) • Richardson (Wood) • Timm (Webber)*

FA PREMIER ACADEMY LEAGUE – UNDER 17s

Neil Bailey's Under 17s had a really close call and could easily have of finished the campaign posing for their team photograph with the FA Premier Academy League Under-17 trophy. Like the under-19s, they had a largely consistent season in their group and at one stage looked more than capable of finishing in top spot. Just five defeats in a 24-match programme wasn't a bad return, but it still left them trailing eventual group winners Liverpool by 17 points. The Anfield lads were in unstoppable form throughout the campaign and finished their programme without a single defeat to record.

At the season's close Bailey's boys found themselves in third place, two points adrift of second-placed Blackburn Rovers and grouped with Southampton, Sheffield Wednesday and Birmingham City in the play-off group section. Wins over the Saints and the Owls plus a point from the trip to Birmingham saw them claim top spot and qualification for the last-eight. They overcame Ipswich Town in the quarter-final before claiming a place in the final via a victory over Leeds United at Thorpe Arch.

Newcastle United had also negotiated a successful route to the final which was staged over two legs at Old Trafford and St James' Park. Newcastle ultimately claimed the prize after winning both games, but there was rarely much to pick between the two sides. The major damage, as far as United were concerned, was done in the first half at Old Trafford when the Magpies swept into a three-goal lead. United did well to claw back two goals after the break but the deficit proved too much and in the second leg Newcastle won 2-0.

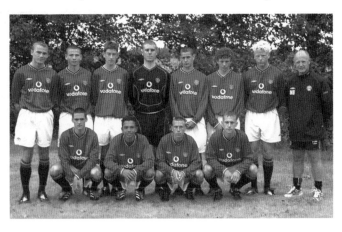

Back row, left to right: Eddie Johnson, Phillip Bardsley, David Jones, James Jowsey, Lee Sims, Ben Collett, Mads Timm, Neil Bailey (coach).
Front row: Danny Byrne, Kieran Richardson, Lee Lawrence, David Poole

names in bold indicate goalscorers

v SOUTHAMPTON (home) • Won: 7-0   Saturday 25 August 2001

Heaton • Picken • Lawrence • Sims • Bardsley • Jones D. • **Timm 2** • **Johnson E. 2** • **Poole 3** • Richardson • Collett
Substitutes: Byrne (Bardsley) • Lee • Eagles • Howard • Nix

v SUNDERLAND (home) • Lost: 1-2   Saturday 8 September 2001

Heaton • Picken • Lawrence • Howard • **Bardsley** • Jones D. • Timm • Byrne • Poole • Calliste • Nix
Substitutes: Nix • Kingsberry • Lee • Leather • Flanagan (Calliste)

v SHEFFIELD UNITED (away) • Won: 6-1   Saturday 15 September 2001

Heaton • Picken • Lawrence • Howard • Bardsley • **Jones D.** • Timm • Byrne • **Poole 2** • **Johnson 2** • Collett
(Tann o.g.)
Substitutes: Eagles (Timm) • Lee • Nix • Eckersley • Flanagan (Johnson)

v NOTTINGHAM FOREST (away) • Won: 6-0   Saturday 29 September 2001

Lee • Picken • Lawrence • Howard • Bardsley • **Jones D.** • Byrne • **Johnson** • **Poole 3** • **Richardson** • Collett
Substitutes: Timm (Poole) • Eagles (Jones D.) • Flanagan (Johnson)

v COVENTRY CITY (away) • Drawn: 1-1   Saturday 6 October 2001

Heaton • Picken • Lawrence • Howard • Bardsley • Jones D. • Byrne • **Johnson** • Calliste • Richardson • Collett
Substitutes: Eagles (Howard) • Lee • Nix (Byrne) • Kouman (Calliste)

v EVERTON (home) • Won: 6-0   Saturday 13 October 2001

Lee • **Picken** • Lawrence • Sims • Bardsley • Jones D. • **Timm** • Byrne • **Poole** • **Johnson 3** • Collett
Substitutes: Eagles • Howard • Eckersley • Kouman

v MANCHESTER CITY (away) • Drawn 2-2   Saturday 20 October 2001

Heaton • Picken • Lawrence • Sims • **Bardsley** • Jones D. • Byrne • Kouman • Timm • **Richardson (pen)** • Collett
Substitutes: Eagles • Eckersley (Timm) • Howard • Kingsberry

v SHEFFIELD WEDNESDAY (home) • Won: 3-2   Tuesday 23 October 2001

Lee • Sims • Lawrence • Howard • Bardsley • Jones D. • Eagles • Timm • Poole • **Richardson 3** • Collett
Substitutes: Eckersley • Calliste (Jones D.) • Port • Jones R.

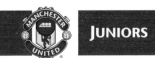

JUNIORS

v WREXHAM (home) • Won: 9-0

Heaton • Picken • Lawrence • Sims • Bardsley • **Timm** • **Eagles** • **Calliste 3** • **Poole 4** • Richardson • Collett
Substitutes: Eckersley (Richardson) • Howard (Bardsley) • Kouman (Timm)

v BLACKBURN ROVERS (away) • Won: 3-1

Heaton • Picken • Lawrence • Sims • Bardsley • Jones D. • Eagles • **Timm** • **Poole** • **Richardson (pen)** • Collett
Substitutes: Eckersley (Collett) • Howard • Calliste • Kouman

v MIDDLESBROUGH (home) • Won: 2-0

Heaton • Picken • Eckersley • Howard • Bardsley • Jones D. • Byrne • Eagles • Poole • **Johnson 2** • Collett
Substitutes: Calliste • Lee • Kouman • Nix

v BOLTON WANDERERS (home) • Won: 4-1

Lee • Picken • Lawrence • Sims • Bardsley • Jones D. • Eagles • **Timm** • Johnson • **Richardson 3** • Collett
Substitutes: Howard • Eckersley • Calliste (Timm) • Kouman

v LIVERPOOL (away) • Lost: 1-5

Lee • Picken • Lawrence • Sims • Howard • **Jones D.** • Timm • Johnson • Poole • Richardson • Collett
Substitutes: Byrne (Richardson) • Eagles (Timm) • Nix • Flanagan

v SHEFFIELD WEDNESDAY (away) • Won: 2-1

Steele • Picken • Eckersley • Nevins • Howard • Jones D. • Byrne • Eagles • **Poole** • **Johnson** • Collett
Substitutes: Flanagan • Lee • Kingsberry • Greenwood • Marsh

v CREWE ALEXANDRA (home) • Drawn: 0-0

Steele • Picken • Lawrence • Howard • Bardsley • Jones D. • Byrne • Eagles • Poole • Johnson • Collett
Substitutes: Eckersley (Lawrence) • Lee • Flanagan • Kouman • Nix

v WREXHAM (away) • Won: 4-1

Lee • Picken • Eckersley • Howard • Bardsley • **Jones D.** • Byrne • **Timm** • **Poole** • **Richardson** • Collett
Substitutes: Eagles • Flanagan • Kouman • Leather • Lawrence

names in bold indicate goalscorers

v BLACKBURN ROVERS (home) • Lost: 1-3 — Saturday 12 January 2002

Lee • Picken • Lawrence • Howard • Bardsley • Jones D. • Byrne • Eagles • Poole • **Johnson** • Collett
Substitutes: Kouman • Nix • Nevins

v MIDDLESBROUGH (away) • Lost: 1-2 — Saturday 19 January 2002

Lee • Picken • Eckersley • Nevins • Howard • Byrne • Timm • Flanagan • **Kouman** • Johnson • Collett
Substitutes: Kingsberry (Nevins) • Port (Kingsberry) • Marsh • Jones R.

v BOLTON WANDERERS (away) • Won: 3-0 — Saturday 26 January 2002

Lee • Picken • Eckersley • Sims • Bardsley • **Byrne** • **Timm** • Eagles • **Blake** • Johnson • Collett
Substitutes: Howard • Flanagan (Johnson) • Port (Timm) • Jones R. • Richardson

v LIVERPOOL (home) • Drawn: 3-3 — Saturday 2 February 2002

Lee • Picken • Eckersley • Nevins • Howard • Jones D. • Byrne • Eagles • **Poole** • **Blake 2** • Collett
Substitutes: Kouman (Jones D.) • Flanagan • Port

v CREWE ALEXANDRA (away) • Drawn: 0-0 — Saturday 9 February 2002

Lee • Picken • Lawrence • Nevins • Howard • Jones D. • Eagles • Byrne • Poole • Johnson • Collett
Substitutes: Kouman • Port • Flanagan • Eckersley

v COVENTRY CITY (home) • Lost: 1-2 — Saturday 16 February 2002

Lee • Picken • Lawrence • Howard • Bardsley • Jones D. • Eagles • Byrne • Poole • **Johnson** • Port
Substitutes: Nevins • Flanagan (Port) • Marsh (Johnson) • Jones R. • Kouman

v EVERTON (away) • Won: 2-0 — Saturday 23 February 2002

Lee • Picken • Lawrence • Sims • Howard • **Jones D.** • Eagles • Byrne • Kouman • **Johnson** • Collett
Substitutes: Poole (Kouman) • Flanagan • Jones R. (Eagles) • Marsh

v MANCHESTER CITY (home) • Drawn: 0-0 — Saturday 9 March 2002

Steele • Nevins • Eckersley • Sims • Howard • Jones D. • Eagles • Byrne • Poole • Johnson • Collett
Substitutes: Kouman • Lee • Nix (Byrne) • Flanagan

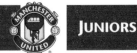

Saturday 16 March 2002   **v SOUTHAMPTON Play-Off (home) • Won: 2-0**

Lee • Picken • **Eckersley** • Sims • Howard • Nix • Eagles • Byrne • Poole • **Calliste** • Collett
Substitutes: Flanagan (Calliste) • Steele • Jones R. • Nevins

Saturday 23 March 2002   **v SHEFFIELD WEDNESDAY Play-Off (home) • Won: 6-0**

Steele • Picken • Eckersley • Sims • Howard • Jones D. • **Eagles** • Byrne • **Poole 2** • Calliste • Collett
(Shirtcliffe o.g.)
*Substitutes: **Flanagan** (Calliste) • Lee • **Port** (Eagles) • Jones R. (Byrne) • Marsh*

Saturday 6 April 2002   **v BIRMINGHAM CITY Play-Off (away) • Drawn: 1-1**

Lee • Picken • Eckersley • Sims • Bardsley • **Jones D.** • Eagles • Byrne • Poole • Calliste • Collett
Substitutes: Jones R. (Byrne) • Port (Jones D.) • Flanagan, Howard

Saturday 20 April 2002   **v IPSWICH TOWN Quarter-Final (home) • Won: 2-1**

Lee • Picken • Lawrence • Sims • Bardsley • Jones D. • Eagles • Collett • Poole • **Johnson** • **Eckersley**
Substitutes: Calliste • Nevins • Flanagan • Jones R.

Saturday 27 April 2002   **v LEEDS UNITED Semi-Final (away) • Won: 2-0**

Lee • Picken • Lawrence • Sims • Bardsley • **Jones D.** • Eagles • Collett • Poole • **Johnson** • Eckersley
Substitutes: Byrne • Heaton • Calliste (Jones D.) • Flanagan • Nevins (Johnson)

Saturday 4 May 2002   **v NEWCASTLE UNITED Final, First Leg (home, at Old Trafford) • Lost: 2-3**

Lee • Picken • Lawrence • Sims • Bardsley • Jones D. • Eagles • Richardson • **Poole** • **Johnson** • Collett
Substitutes: Byrne (Eagles) • Heaton • Eckersley • Calliste • Nevins

Monday 13 April 2002   **v NEWCASTLE UNITED Final, Second Leg (away, at St James' Park) • Lost: 0-2**

Steele • Byrne • Lawrence • Sims • Bardsley • Jones D. • Timm • Richardson • Poole • Johnson • Collett
Substitutes: Marsh (Byrne) • Simpson (Timm)

UNDER 17s APPEARANCES

Name	Appearances (as sub)	Name	Appearances (as sub)
COLLETT • Ben	29	RICHARDSON • Kieran	12
PICKEN • Philip	28	HEATON • Tom	8
JONES • David	27	CALLISTE • Ramon	6 (3)
POOLE • David	25 (1)	NEVINS • Adrian	5 (1)
BYRNE • Danny	22 (3)	STEELE • Luke	5
BARDSLEY • Phillip	22	KOUMAN • Amadou	3 (3)
JOHNSON • Eddie	21	NIX • Kyle	2 (2)
LAWRENCE • Lee	21	BLAKE • Sylvan	2
EAGLES • Christopher	20 (4)	FLANAGAN • Callum	1 (7)
HOWARD • Mark	19	PORT • Graeme	1 (4)
LEE • Tommy	18	JONES • Richard	0 (3)
SIMS • Lee	18	MARSH • Philip	0 (2)
TIMM • Mads	14	KINGSBERRY • Chris	0 (1)
ECKERSLEY • Adam	12 (4)	SIMPSON • Danny	0 (1)

GOALSCORERS

Name	Goals
JOHNSON • Eddie	21
POOLE • David	20
TIMM • Mads	8
JONES • David	7
RICHARDSON • Kieran	7
CALLISTE • Ramon	4
BLAKE • Sylvain	3
BARDSLEY • Phillip	2
EAGLES • Christopher	2
ECKERSLEY • Adam	2
BYRNE • Danny	1
FLANAGAN • Callum	1
PICKEN • Philip	1
PORT • Graeme	1
KOUMAN • Amadou	1

Own Goals

SHIRTCLIFFE • Chris (Sheffield Wednesday)	1 o.g.
TANN • Lee (Sheffield United)	1 o.g.

FA PREMIER ACADEMY LEAGUE UNDER 17s

GROUP C FINAL TABLE 2001-02

	P	W	D	L	F	A	Pts
Liverpool	24	19	5	0	75	16	62
Blackburn Rovers	24	13	8	3	53	21	47
MANCHESTER UNITED	24	13	6	5	68	27	45
Coventry City	24	10	6	8	37	38	36
Crewe Alexandra	24	10	5	9	28	36	35
Manchester City	24	7	9	8	37	40	30
Bolton Wanderers	24	5	2	17	33	60	17
Everton	24	4	4	16	18	47	16
Wrexham	24	2	5	17	19	71	11

FA PREMIER ACADEMY LEAGUE UNDER 17s PLAY–OFFS

GROUP TWO FINAL TABLE 2001-02

	P	W	D	L	F	A	Pts
MANCHESTER UNITED	3	2	1	0	9	1	7
Birmingham City	3	1	1	1	3	3	4
Southampton	3	1	0	2	1	3	3
Sheffield Wednesday	3	1	0	2	2	8	3

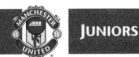

COCA-COLA CUP 15TH JUNIOR TOURNAMENT – OLPE, GERMANY

Saturday 18 August 2001   **v SpVg OLPE (Germany) Group B • Drawn: 0-0**

Lee • Picken • Lawrence • Sims • Bardsley • Jones • Timm • Byrne • Poole • Johnson • Collett
Substitutes: Eagles (Byrne) • Calliste (Poole)

Saturday 18 August 2001   **v MALMO FF (Sweden) Group B • Won: 2-1**

Lee • Picken • Lawrence • Sims • Bardsley • **Jones** • Timm • Byrne • Poole • **Calliste** • Collett
Substitutes: Eagles (Jones) • Kouman (Calliste)

Sunday 19 August 2001   **v VfL BOCHUM (Germany) Group B • Lost : 1-2**

Lee • Picken • Lawrence • Sims • Bardsley • Jones • Timm • Byrne • **Poole** • Johnson • Collett

Sunday 19 August 2001   **v MIDDLESBROUGH (England) Third/Fourth Place Play-Off • Lost: 0-1**

Heaton • Eagles • Eckersley • Sims • Bardsley • Jones • Timm • Byrne • Kouman • Calliste • Collett

TOURNAMENT SQUAD

Phillip BARDSLEY	Christopher EAGLES	David JONES	Phil PICKEN
Danny BYRNE	Adam ECKERSLEY	Amadou KOUMAN	David POOLE
Ramon CALLISTE	Tom HEATON	Lee LAWRENCE	Lee SIMS
Ben COLLETT	Eddie JOHNSON	Tommy LEE	Mads TIMM

FRIENDLIES

Saturday 4 August 2001   **v FLEETWOOD FREEPORT (away) • Won: 6-1**

Jowsey • Clegg S. • **Taylor K.** • Sims • Cogger • Byrne • Timm • Johnson E. • **Poole 2** • Richardson • Collett
*Substitutes: Taylor A. (Cogger) • Heaton • Mooniaruck (Taylor K.) • Humphreys (Richardson) • **Heath 3** (Johnson E.)*

Friday 10 August 2001   **v SAN DIEGO NOMADS (United States of America) (home) • Won: 6-1**

Heaton • Picken • Lawrence • Sims • Bardsley • **Jones D.** • **Timm** • **Johnson E.** • Poole • **Richardson** • **Collett**
*Substitutes: Fox (Richardson) • Lee (Heaton) • **Calliste** (Johnson E.) • Kouman (Poole) • Kingsberry (Timm) • Eckersley (Lawrence)*

Saturday 1 September 2001   **v OMAN (home) • Won: 6-1**

Moran • Sims • Lawrence • **Taylor K.** • **Cogger** • Jones D. • Heath • **Johnson 2** • **Poole** • **Richardson** • Collett
Substitutes: Fox (Heath) • Curran, trialist (Moran) • Bardsley (Jones D.) • Camilleri, trialist (Johnson)

NIVEA UNDER 17s JUNIOR FOOTBALL TOURNAMENT
– BLUDENZ, AUSTRIA

v JAPAN Group B • Drawn: 0-0   Saturday 30 March 2002

Lee • Picken • Eckersley • Howard • Bardsley • Jones • Port • Eagles • Flanagan • Calliste • White

v AUSTRIA Group B • Won: 1-0   Sunday 31 March 2002

Lee • Picken • Eckersley • Howard • Bardsley • Jones • Port • Eagles • Flanagan • Calliste • **Kouman**
Substitutes: Marsh (Flanagan) • Simpson (Jones)

v DINAMO ZAGREB (Croatia) • Drawn: 1-1   Sunday 31 March 2002

Lee • Simpson • Hogg • Howard • Bardsley • White • Port • Eagles • Flanagan • Marsh • Kouman
*Substitutes: Picken (Kouman) • Eckersley (White) • **Calliste** (Flanagan) • Heaton (Marsh)*

v LIVERPOOL (England) Semi-Final • Lost: 0-1   Monday 1 April 2002

Lee • Picken • Eckersley • Howard • Bardsley • Jones • Port • Eagles • Hogg • Calliste • Kouman
Substitute: Flanagan (Hogg)

v DINAMO ZAGREB (Croatia) Third/Fourth Place Play-Off • Lost: 0-1   Monday 1 April 2002

Lee • Picken • Eckersley • Howard • Bardsley • Jones • Simpson • Eagles • Flanagan • Marsh • White
Substitutes: Calliste (Marsh) • Kouman (White)

TOURNAMENT SQUAD

Phillip BARDSLEY	Richard JONES
Ramon CALLISTE	Amadou KOUMAN
Christopher EAGLES	Tom LEE
Adam ECKERSLEY	Philip MARSH
Callum FLANAGAN	Philip PICKEN
Tom HEATON	Graeme PORT
Stephen HOGG	Danny SIMPSON
Mark HOWARD	Christopher WHITE

NORTHERN IRELAND MILK CUP
INTERNATIONAL YOUTH TOURNAMENT 2001 (UNDER 16s)

Monday 23 July 2001   **v COUNTY TYRONE (Northern Ireland) Qualifying • Won: 4-0**

Heaton • Picken • Lawrence • Sims • **Poole** • Jones • Byrne • **Johnson** • **Timm** • **Richardson** • Collett
Substitutes: Fox (Poole) • Eckersley (Lawrence) • Howard (Sims) • Nevins (Picken) • Kingsberry (Johnson)

Tuesday 24 July 2001   **v ICHIRITSU FUNABASHI (Japan) Qualifying • Drawn: 2-2**

Heaton • Picken • Lawrence • Sims • Poole • Jones • Byrne • **Johnson** • Timm • **Richardson (pen)** • Collett
Substitute: Howard (Picken)

Wednesday 25 July 2001   **v CD PALESTINO (Chile) Quarter-Final • Drawn: 1-1***

Heaton • Poole • Lawrence • Sims • Bardsley • Jones • Byrne • Johnson • Timm • **Richardson (pen)** • Collett
Substitutes: Eckersley (Timm) • Kingsberry (Byrne)
* **Won on penalties**. *Penalty-scorers:* Bardsley • Richardson • Poole • Collett

Thursday 26 July 2001   **v BOTAFOGO (Brazil) Semi-Final • Won: 1-0**

Heaton • Picken • Lawrence • Sims • Bardsley • Kingsberry • Poole • Johnson • Fox • **Richardson (pen)** • Collett
Substitute: Eckersley (Johnson)

Friday 27 July 2001   **v PARAGUAY Final • Lost: 0-6**

Heaton • Picken • Lawrence • Sims • Bardsley • Poole • Byrne • Johnson • Timm • Richardson • Collett
Substitute: Howard (Byrne)

TOURNAMENT SQUAD

Phil BARDSLEY	Chris KINGSBERRY
Danny BYRNE	Lee LAWRENCE
Ben COLLETT	Tommy LEE
Adam ECKERSLEY	Adrian NEVINS
Mark FOX	Phil PICKEN
Tom HEATON	David POOLE
Mark HOWARD	Kieran RICHARDSON
Eddie JOHNSON	Lee SIMS
David JONES	Mads TIMM

8TH INTERNATIONAL FRIENDSHIP YOUTH TOURNAMENT – VENICE, ITALY

v AC TORINO (Italy) Group C • Lost: 0-2 — Thursday 30 August 2001

Heaton • Picken • Eckersley • Leather • Howard • Port • Kingsberry • Eagles • Kouman • Calliste • Nix

v UDINESE (Italy) Group C • Won: 1-0 — Friday 31 August 2001

Lee • Picken • Eckersley • Leather • Howard • Jones • Kingsberry • **Eagles** • Flanagan • Calliste • Nix

Substitutes: Greenwood (Eagles) • White (Kingsberry)

v US SANVITESE (Italy) Group C • Won: 8-1 — Friday 31 August 2001

Heaton • **Picken** • **Eckersley** • Leather • Howard • Jones • Kingsberry • Greenwood • **Kouman** • **Flanagan** • **Nix**

*Substitutes: Port (Picken) • Fox (Jones) • **Marsh 3** (Flanagan) • White (Nix)*

v EINTRACHT FRANKFURT (Germany) Quarter-Final • Drawn: 2-2* — Saturday 1 September 2001

Heaton • Picken • Eckersley • Leather • Howard • Jones • Kingsberry • Eagles • **Flanagan** • **Calliste** • Nix

Substitutes: Kouman (Flanagan) • Greenwood (Kingsberry)

* **Lost 1-2 on penalties.** *Penalty-scorer: Leather*

v SPARTAK MOSCOW (Russia) Fifth/Sixth Place Play-Off • Won: 5-0 — Sunday 2 September 2001

Lee • Picken • Eckersley • Leather • Howard • Jones • Port • **Eagles** • **Flanagan** • **Calliste** • White

*Substitutes: Kouman (Calliste) • **Marsh 2** (Flanagan)*

TOURNAMENT SQUAD

Ramon CALLISTE	Chris KINGSBERRY
Christopher EAGLES	Amadou KOUMAN
Adam ECKERSLEY	Wayne LEATHER
Callum FLANAGAN	Tommy LEE
Mark FOX	Philip MARSH
Ross GREENWOOD	Kyle NIX
Tom HEATON	Philip PICKEN
Mark HOWARD	Graeme PORT
Reece JONES	Chris WHITE

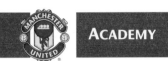

MANCHESTER UNITED ACADEMY – UNDER 16s/15s

Sunday 26 August 2001   **v ROTHERHAM UNITED (home) • Won: 3-1**

Lee • Nevins • White • Leather • Howard • Jones (Reece) • Jones (Richard) • Eagles • Flanagan • Abdillahi • Nix
Substitutes: Marsh • Calliste

Sunday 2 September 2001   **v STOKE CITY (home) • Won: 4-2**

Lee • Greenwood • Eckersley • Hogg • Leather • Camilleri • Kingsberry • Jones (Reece) • Flanagan • Kouman • White
Substitutes: Jones (Richard) • Marsh

Sunday 16 September 2001   **v LIVERPOOL (home) • Won: 1-0**

Lee • Greenwood • Eckersley • White • Nevins • Jones (Reece) • Jones (Richard) • Eagles • Flanagan • Calliste • Nix
Substitute: Marsh

Sunday 23 September 2001   **v SHEFFIELD WEDNESDAY (away) • Won: 2-1**

Lee • Greenwood • Eckersley • White • Howard • Jones (Reece) • Jones (Richard) • Eagles • Flanagan • Kouman • Nix
Substitute: Marsh

Sunday 7 October 2001   **v CREWE ALEXANDRA (home) • Won: 3-0**

Lee • Greenwood • Eckersley • Nevins • Leather • Jones (Reece) • Kingsberry • Eagles • Flanagan • Kouman • Nix
Substitutes: Marsh • White • Port

Sunday 21 October 2001   **v BOLTON WANDERERS (home) • Won: 6-0**

Lee • Greenwood • Nevins • Leather • Howard • Jones (Reece) • Kingsberry • Eagles • Flanagan • Marsh • White
Substitutes: Nix • Jones (Richard) • Port • Eckersley

Sunday 28 October 2001   **v MANCHESTER CITY (away) • Lost: 0-4**

Allan • Greenwood • Eckersley • Nevins • Howard • Jones (Reece) • Kingsberry • Port • Flanagan • Kouman • White
Substitutes: Jones (Richard) • Leather • Marsh

Sunday 4 November 2001   **v BIRMINGHAM CITY (home) • Won: 2-0**

Lee • Greenwood • Eckersley • Nevins • Leather • Nix • Kingsberry • Kouman • Flanagan • Calliste • Port
Substitutes: Jones (Reece) • Howard • Marsh

v BLACKBURN ROVERS (home) • Won: 2-0 — Sunday 11 November 2001

Lee • Greenwood • Nix • Jones (Richard) • Flanagan • Jones (Reece) • Kingsberry • Kouman • Marsh • Calliste • Port

v STOKE CITY (home) • Won: 3-1 — Wednesday 14 November 2001

Lee • Jones (Reece) • White • Eckersley • Howard • Jones (Richard) • Kingsberry • Kouman • Flanagan • Calliste • Port
Substitutes: Marsh • Uccello • Eagles • Simpson • Picken

v HUDDERSFIELD TOWN (away) • Won: 4-0 — Sunday 18 November 2001

Lee • Greenwood • Eckersley • Nevins • Howard • Jones (Reece) • Kingsberry • Kouman • Flanagan • Calliste • Nix
Substitutes: Jones (Richard) • Marsh • White • Uccello

v LIVERPOOL (away) • Won: 2-0 — Wednesday 28 November 2001

Lee • Greenwood • Eckersley • Nevins • Howard • Jones (Reece) • Picken • Eagles • Flanagan • Kouman • Kingsberry
Substitutes: Marsh • White

v BARNSLEY (home) • Won: 6-0 — Sunday 9 December 2001

Lee • Jones (Richard) • Eckersley • Nevins • Leather • Nix • Port • Jones (Reece) • Flanagan • Kouman • Kingsberry
Substitutes: Marsh • Fitzsimmons

v HUDDERSFIELD TOWN (home) • Won: 3-2 — Sunday 16 December 2001

Fitzsimmons • Jones (Richard) • Nix • Nevins • Leather • Jones (Reece) • Kingsberry • Eagles • Flanagan • Kouman • Port
Substitutes: Marsh • Lee

v LEICESTER CITY (away) • Won: 7-2 — Sunday 13 January 2002

Lee • Greenwood • Nix • Nevins • Leather • Jones (Reece) • Kingsberry • Port • Flanagan • Kouman • White
Substitutes: Jones (Richard) • Marsh • Hogg

v EVERTON (away) • Drawn: 0-0 — Wednesday 30 January 2002

Robinson • Nevins • White • Leather • Howard • Jones (Richard) • Kingsberry • Kouman • Flanagan • Blake • Port
Substitutes: Eagles • Eckersley • Picken • Hogg

ACADEMY

v SHEFFIELD WEDNESDAY (home) • Won: 3-0

Robinson • Simpson • Nix • Hogg • Eckersley • Jones (Richard) • Kingsberry • Kouman • Flanagan • Marsh • Port
Substitutes: Howard • Lee • Calliste

v HUDDERSFIELD TOWN (home) • Won: 5-1

Robinson • Simpson • White • Howard • Nevins • Jones (Richard) • Kingsberry • Port • Flanagan • Calliste • Nix
Substitutes: Fox • Lee • Marsh • Eagles • Kouman

v NOTTINGHAM FOREST (away) • Lost: 1-2

Lee • Picken • Nix • Nevins • Howard • Jones (Richard) • Calliste • Eagles • Flanagan • Kouman • Port
Substitutes: Fox • Marsh

v BOLTON WANDERERS (away) • Won: 3-2

Lee • Simpson • Nix • Jones (Richard) • Nevins • Kouman • Marsh • Flanagan • Fox • Calliste • Port
Substitutes: Eckersley • Howard • Eagles

v BLACKBURN ROVERS (away) • Won: 1-0

Lee • Ward • Hogg • Nevins • Howard • Jones (Richard) • Simpson • Eagles • Flanagan • Marsh • Port
Substitutes: Calliste • Eckersley

v LIVERPOOL (away) • Won: 1-0

Lee • Simpson • Eckersley • Picken • Nevins • Jones (Richard) • Eagles • Martin • Marsh • Calliste • Port
Substitute: Flanagan

v HUDDERSFIELD TOWN (home) • Won: 7-1

Lee • Picken • Eckersley • Nevins • Hogg • Martin • Eagles • Jones (Richard) • Flanagan • Calliste • Port
Substitutes: Marsh • Simpson

MANCHESTER UNITED ACADEMY – UNDER 14s

v STOKE CITY (home) • Won: 3-2 — Sunday 2 September 2001

Daniels • Simpson • Baker • Lea • Lee • Baguley • Campbell • **Parillon 2** • Burns • Parrott • Moore

*Substitutes: **Farrelly** • Shawcross • Howard*

v EVERTON (away) • Lost: 2-3 — Sunday 9 September 2001

Daniels • Baker • Lea • Lee • Simpson • Howard • **Parillon** • **Campbell** • Burns • Baguley • Moore

Substitutes: Farrelly • Shawcross

v LIVERPOOL (away) • Won: 2-0 — Sunday 16 September 2001

Daniels • Baker • Lea • Lee • Simpson • Howard • **Parillon** • Campbell • Burns • Baguley • Moore

*Substitutes: Farrelly • **Parrott** • Shawcross*

v SHEFFIELD WEDNESDAY (home) • Won: 5-0 — Sunday 23 September 2001

Daniels • Baker • Lea • Lee • Shawcross • Simpson • **Parillon** • Campbell • Burns • **Baguley 2** • Farrelly

(1 o.g.)

*Substitutes: **Parrott** • Moore • Howard*

v CREWE ALEXANDRA (away) • Drawn: 2-2 — Sunday 7 October 2001

Daniels • Baker • Lea • Lee • Simpson • Howard • Parillon • **Campbell** • Burns • **Baguley** • Moore

Substitutes: Shawcross • Yarwood • Stott

v LEEDS UNITED (away) • Won: 2-1 — Sunday 14 October 2001

Daniels • Baker • Lea • Lee • Simpson • Shawcross • Parillon • **Campbell** • Burns • Baguley • Moore

*Substitutes: Howard • Yarwood • **Stott***

v LIVERPOOL (away) • Won: 4-1 — Tuesday 16 October 2001

Daniels • Baker • Lea • **Lee 3** • Simpson • Howard • Parillon • Campbell • Yarwood • Baguley • Moore

*Substitutes: **Burns** • Shawcross • Stott*

v BOLTON WANDERERS (home) • Won: 11-0 — Sunday 21 October 2001

Daniels • Baker • Lea • Shawcross • Simpson • **Howard** • **Brandy** • **Stott** • **Yarwood 2** • **Baguley** • Burns

*Substitutes: **Lee** • **Parillon 2** • **Campbell 2***

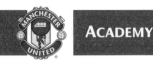

ACADEMY

v MANCHESTER CITY (away) • Lost: 0-4

Daniels • Baker • Lea • Lee • Simpson • Howard • Parillon • Campbell • Yarwood • Baguley • Burns
Substitutes: Shawcross • Moore • Stott • Farrelly

v BIRMINGHAM CITY (away) • Lost: 3-5

Allen • Baker • Lea • **Lee** • Simpson • Howard • Parillon • Campbell • Yarwood • Baguley • **Burns 2**
Substitutes: Shawcross • Daniels • Moore • Parrott

v EVERTON (away) • Won: 1-0

Daniels • Baker • Lea • Lee • Simpson • Shawcross • Parillon • Campbell • Yarwood • **Burns** • Moore
Substitutes: Howard • Allen • Parrott • Baguley

v BLACKBURN ROVERS (away) • Won: 2-1

Daniels • Baker • Lea • Lee • **Simpson** • Howard • Parillon • **Campbell** • Burns • Baguley • Moore
Substitutes: Shawcross • Parrott • Yarwood

v HUDDERSFIELD TOWN (home) • Won: 4-1

Daniels • Baker • Lea • Lee • Shawcross • **Howard** • **Parillon** • **Campbell 2** • Parrot • Baguley • Moore
Substitutes: Burns • Simpson

v WREXHAM (home) • Won: 6-1

Daniels • Baker • Lea • **Lee** • Simpson • Howard • **Parillon 4** • **Campbell** • Parrott • Baguley • Burns
Substitutes: Moore • Shawcross

v QUEENSLAND STATE SOCCER FEDERATION (Australia) (home) • Drawn: 1-1

Daniels • Baker • Lea • Lee • Simpson • Parillon • Campbell • **Marsh** • Parrot • Baguley • Moore
Substitutes: Burns • Allan • Shawcross

v BARNSLEY (home) • Drawn: 2-2

Allan • Baker • Lea • Lee • Simpson • Shawcross • **Campbell** • Parillon • **Parrott** • Baguley • Moore
Substitutes: Burns • Daniels • Howard

names in bold indicate goalscorers

v SUNDERLAND (home) • Won: 2-0 — Sunday 16 December 2001

Daniels • Simpson • Lea • Lee • Shawcross • **Howard** • Parillon • **Baker** • Parrott • Baguley • Burns

Substitutes: Campbell • Allan • Moore

v LIVERPOOL (home) • Drawn: 2-2 — Sunday 13 January 2002

Daniels • Baker • Lea • Lee • Shawcross • Simpson • **Parillon** • Campbell • Parrott • Baguley • Burns

(1 o.g.)

Substitutes: Howard • Moore

v STOKE CITY (home) • Won: 5-1 — Sunday 20 January 2002

Daniels • Baker • Lea • Lee • Simpson • **Hewson** • Parillon • **Brandy** • **Burns 2** • **Baguley** • Moore

Substitute: Heath

v LIVERPOOL (away) • Won: 3-0 — Sunday 3 February 2002

Daniels • Baker • Lea • Lee • Simpson • Booth • Parillon • **Campbell** • **Burns** • Nix • Shawcross

*Substitutes: Baguley • Rhodes • Moore • Howard • **Parrott***

v SHEFFIELD WEDNESDAY (away) • Lost: 0-1 — Sunday 10 February 2002

Rhodes • Baker • Lea • Lee • Shawcross • Howard • Booth • Nix • Parrott • Baguley • Moore

Substitute: Campbell • Daniels • Parillon • Burns

v SUNDERLAND (away) • Lost: 1-2 — Sunday 17 February 2002

Daniels • Baker • Howard • **Lee** • Simpson • Shawcross • Campbell • Parillon • Burns • Baguley • Nix

Substitute: Moore

v CREWE ALEXANDRA (home) • Lost: 1-3 — Sunday 24 February 2002

Daniels • Baker • Lea • **Lee** • Shawcross • Howard • Parillon • Campbell • Burns • Baguley • Nix

Substitutes: Moore • Brandy • Hewson

v LEEDS UNITED (away) • Lost: 1-3 — Sunday 3 March 2002

Daniels • Baker • Lea • Lee • Simpson • Shawcross • Campbell • **Parillon** • Burns • Baguley • Howard

Substitutes: Moore • Rhodes • Parrott

ACADEMY

v BOLTON WANDERERS (away) • Lost: 0-1

Daniels • Baker • Lea • Lee • Booth • Howard • Campbell • Parillon • Burns • Baguley • Moore
Substitute: Parrott

v MANCHESTER CITY (home) • Won: 3-2

Daniels • Simpson • Drinkwater • **Lee** • Shawcross • Lea • Booth • **Campbell 2** • Burns • Parrott • Howard
Substitutes: Baguley • Baker • Moore • Nix

v BIRMINGHAM CITY (home) • Won: 2-1

Rhodes • Baker • Lee • Simpson • Shawcross • Booth • Parillon • **Campbell** • **Burns** • Baguley • Moore
Substitutes: Lea • Daniels • Howard • Drinkwater

v NORWICH CITY (away) • Won: 1-0

Daniels • Baker • Drinkwater • Lee • Shawcross • Lea • Parillon • **Campbell** • Burns • Baguley • Booth
Substitutes: Nix • Howard • Parrott • Moore • Heath

v BLACKBURN ROVERS (home) • Lost: 0-1

Daniels • Baker • Lea • Lee • Shawcross • Howard • Campbell • Parillon • Burns • Nix • Drinkwater
Substitutes: Baguley • Booth • Moore

v HUDDERSFIELD TOWN (away) • Won: 3-1

Daniels • Lee • Lea • Shawcross • Burns • Howard • **Parillon** • **Campbell** • **Parrott** • Baguley • Moore
Substitute: Crump

v WREXHAM (away) • Drawn: 1-1

Daniels • Baker • Lea • Lee • Burns • Moore • Parillon • **Campbell** • Burns • Baguley • Tracey
Substitutes: Booth • Crump

v BARNSLEY (away) • Lost: 0-1

Daniels • Simpson • Shawcross • Lee • Lea • Booth • Parillon • Campbell • Burns • Baguley • Moore
Substitutes: Baker • Crump • Parrott

v EVERTON (home) • Won: 1-0

Crump • Baker • Lea • Simpson • Shawcross • Booth • Parillon • Lee • Brandy • Baguley • Heath
*Substitutes: Burns • **Howard** • Hewson • Moore*

MANCHESTER UNITED ACADEMY – UNDER 13s

v STOKE CITY (home) • Won: 6-2 Sunday 2 September 2001

Ingram-Hughes • Cleverley • Drinkwater • Chester • Kendrick • Hewson • Coleman • Owens • Brandy • Hanson • Rowe T.
Substitutes: Eckersley • Rowe D. • Thompson

v EVERTON (home) • Lost: 2-3 Sunday 9 September 2001

Amos • Eckersley • Drinkwater • Chester • Kendrick • Hewson • Thompson • Rowe D. • Brandy • Hanson • Rowe T.
Substitutes: Cleverley • Owens • Coleman

v LIVERPOOL (home) • Lost: 2-4 Sunday 16 September 2001

Amos • Cleverley • Drinkwater • Chester • Kendrick • Hewson • Thompson • Owens • Brandy • Hanson • Heath
Substitutes: Eckersley • Rowe T. • Rowe D. • Coleman

v SHEFFIELD WEDNESDAY (away) • Drawn: 3-3 Sunday 23 September 2001

Amos • Cleverley • Drinkwater • Chester • Kendrick • Hewson • Eckersley • Heath • Brandy • Rowe D. • Rowe T.
Substitutes: Owens • Thompson • Hanson • Coleman

v CREWE ALEXANDRA (home) • Won: 4-3 Sunday 7 October 2001

Ingram-Hughes • Cleverley • Drinkwater • Chester • Hewson • Owens • Eckersley • Heath • Rowe D. • Coleman • Thompson
Substitutes: Brandy • Hanson

v LEEDS UNITED (away) • Won: 3-2 Sunday 14 October 2001

Amos • Cleverley • Drinkwater • Heath • Chester • Hewson • Eckersley • Rowe D. • Brandy • Hanson • Owens
Substitute: Coleman

v BOLTON WANDERERS (away) • Won: 3-1 Sunday 21 October 2001

Ingram-Hughes • Cleverley • Drinkwater • Chester • Kendrick • Rowe D. • Heath • Eckersley • Thompson • Hanson • Owens
Substitute: Coleman

v MANCHESTER CITY (home) • Won: 5-1 Sunday 28 October 2001

Ingram-Hughes • Cleverley • Drinkwater • Chester • Kendrick • Hewson • Eckersley • Heath • Hanson • Brandy • Owens
Substitutes: Rowe D. • Thompson • Rowe T. • Coleman

Sunday 4 November 2001   **v BIRMINGHAM CITY (home) • Won: 1-0**

Amos • Cleverley • Drinkwater • Chester • Kendrick • Hewson • Eckersley • Heath • Hanson • Brandy • Owens
Substitutes: Rowe T. • Coleman • Rowe D. • Thompson

Sunday 11 November 2001   **v BLACKBURN ROVERS (home) • Drawn: 3-3**

Amos • Cleverley • Drinkwater • Chester • Kendrick • Hewson • Thompson • Heath • Rowe • Coleman • Owens
Substitutes: Brandy • Hanson • Eckersley

Sunday 18 November 2001   **v HUDDERSFIELD TOWN (away) • Won: 7-2**

Amos • Cleverley • Drinkwater • Chester • Kendrick • Hewson • Eckersley • Thompson • Rowe D. • Coleman • Owens
Substitutes: Hanson • Brandy

Sunday 25 November 2001   **v WREXHAM (away) • Drawn: 0-0**

Amos • Cleverley • Eckersley • Chester • Drinkwater • Hewson • Thompson • Rowe D. • Brandy • Coleman • Rowe T.

Sunday 9 December 2001   **v BARNSLEY (away) • Won: 12-1**

Ingram-Hughes • Cleverley • Drinkwater • Chester • Kendrick • Hewson • Eckersley • Heath • Brandy • Rowe D. • Rowe T.
Substitutes: Coleman • Thompson

Sunday 16 December 2001   **v SUNDERLAND (away) • Won: 6-1**

Ingram-Hughes • Cleverley • Drinkwater • Kendrick • Chester • Hewson • Thompson • Heath • Brandy • Coleman • Rowe T.
Substitute: Rowe D.

Sunday 20 January 2002   **v STOKE CITY (away) • Won: 1-0**

Amos • Cleverley • Drinkwater • Williams • Chester • Kendrick • Thompson • Rowe D. • Coleman • Hanson • Rowe T.
Substitutes: Owens • Eckersley

Sunday 27 January 2002   **v EVERTON (home) • Won: 2-0**

Amos • Eckersley • Drinkwater • Heath • Chester • Hewson • Rowe D. • Owens • Brandy • Hanson • Rowe T.

v LIVERPOOL (home) • Lost: 3-5 — Sunday 3 February 2002

Amos • Cleverley • Drinkwater • Chester • Kendrick • Hewson • Eckersley • Heath • Brandy • Coleman • Owens

Substitutes: Hanson • Rowe T. • Thompson • Rowe D.

v SHEFFIELD WEDNESDAY (home) • Won: 3-2 — Sunday 10 February 2002

Amos • Eckersley • Drinkwater • Chester • Kendrick • Hewson • Thompson • Owens • Rowe D. • Brandy • Rowe T.

Substitutes: Coleman • Hanson • Cleverley

v SUNDERLAND (home) • Won: 5-1 — Sunday 17 February 2002

Amos • Eckersley • Drinkwater • Chester • Kendrick • Hewson • Thompson • Owens • Coleman • Hanson • Rowe T.

Substitutes: Brandy • Cleverley

v LEEDS UNITED (home) • Lost: 2-3 — Sunday 3 March 2002

Amos • Kendrick • Drinkwater • Chester • Heath • Hewson • Eckersley • Owens • Brandy • Rowe D. • Rowe T.

Substitutes: Cleverley • Hanson • Coleman • Thompson

v BOLTON WANDERERS (home) • Lost: 1-2 — Sunday 10 March 2002

Rhodes • Cleverley • Drinkwater • Chester • Kendrick • Hewson • Thompson • Heath • Brandy • Coleman • Rowe T.

Substitutes: Rowe D. • Eckersley • Hanson • Owens

v MANCHESTER CITY (away) • Won: 3-0 — Sunday 17 March 2002

Rhodes • Cleverley • Heath • Chester • Kendrick • Hewson • Eckersley • Owens • Brandy • Coleman • Rowe T.

Substitutes: Rowe D. • Hansen • Thompson

v BIRMINGHAM CITY (away) • Lost: 4-7 — Sunday 24 March 2002

Amos • Eckersley • Heath • Chester • Kendrick • Hewson • Thompson • Owens • Rowe D. • Hanson • Rowe T.

Substitutes: Brandy • Coleman • Cleverley

v BLACKBURN ROVERS (away) • Won: 2-1 — Sunday 7 April 2002

Amos • Eckersley • Heath • Chester • Kendrick • Rowe D. • Cleverley • Owens • Brandy • Coleman • Rowe T.

Substitute: Thompson • Hanson

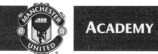
Sunday 14 April 2002

v HUDDERSFIELD TOWN (home) • Won: 3-1

Amos • Cleverley • Eckersley • Chester • Kendrick • Hewson • Thompson • Owens • Rowe T. • Hanson • Heath
Substitute: Rowe D.

Sunday 21 April 2002

v WREXHAM (home) • Won: 9-0

Amos • Eckersley • Cleverley • Chester • Kendrick • Hewson • Thompson • Owens • Brandy • Rowe T. • Heath
Substitutes: Hanson • Coleman • Rowe D.

Sunday 28 April 2002

v BARNSLEY (home) • Drawn: 0-0

Amos • Eckersley • Cleverley • Chester • Kendrick • Hewson • Thompson • Owens • Rowe • Hanson • Heath
Substitutes: Brandy • Rowe T. • Coleman

UNDER 12s

SQUAD

Benjamin AMOS
Nicholas BLACKMAN
Antonio BRYAN
Jacob BUTTERFIELD
Jonathan CROMPTON
James DERBYSHIRE
Daniel DRINKWATER
Dominic LILLIE

Jay McGARVEY
Thomas MELLOR
Alex SKIDMORE
Gregory WILKINSON

UNDER 11s

SQUAD

Philip BROWN
Kristopher DICKINSON
Joseph DUDGEON
Shaun JOHNSON
Jacob LAWLOR
Ben MARSHALL
Thomas MINNS
Oliver NORWOOD

Daniel WELBECK
David WILLIAMS
Matthew WILLIAMS

UNDER 10s

SQUAD

Nicholas AJOSEN
Peter BIRCH
Reece BROWN
Brad BYRNE
Thomas DAVIES
Mark DUNCAN
Peter GREGSON
Sam ILLINGWORTH

William MELLOR
Justin PICKERING
Michael POTTS
Matthew REAM

UNDER 9s

SQUAD

Thomas BENTHAM
Larnell COLE
Daniel COULTHARD
Zach FLYNN
Luke GIVERIN
Jake HARRISON
Nicholas JACKSON
Jesse LINGARD

Jay LYNCH
David MELLOR
Ravel MORRISON
Kieran O'BOYLE
Joshua PRITCHARD
Thomas THORPE
Ryan TUNNICLIFFE

DORINT CUP YOUTH TOURNAMENT – RUESSELSHEIM, GERMANY

v WERDER BREMEN (Germany) Group Stage • Drawn: 0-0   Saturday 18 May 2002

Daniels • Simpson • Lea • Lee • Shawcross • Howard • Parillon • Campbell • Burns • Baguley • Moore

v JSG MORLENBACH (Germany) Group Stage • Won: 2-0   Saturday 18 May 2002

Daniels • Simpson • Baker • Lea • Shawcross • **Hewson** • Parillon • Campbell • **Booth** • Heath • Parrott

v TV MECKELFELD (Germany) Group Stage • Won: 4-0   Saturday 18 May 2002

Daniels • Simpson • Baker • **Lee 2** • Moore • Howard • Parillon • Campbell • **Burns** • Baguley • **Parrott**
Substitutes: Hewson (Parillon) • Heath (Simpson) • Booth (Campbell)

v JSG MORLENBACH (Germany) Last Sixteen • Won: 4-0   Sunday 19 May 2002

Daniels • Simpson • **Lea** • Lee • Shawcross • Baker • Parillon • Campbell • Moore • Baguley • Parrott
*Substitutes: **Burns** (Parillon) • Booth (Baguley) • Hewson (Lee) • Howard (Shawcross) • **Heath 2** (Moore)*

v KAISERSLAUTERN (Germany) • Drawn: 0-0*   Monday 20 May 2002

Daniels • Simpson • Lea • Lee • Shawcross • Baker • Parillon • Campbell • Moore • Baguley • Parrott
Substitutes: Hewson (Baker) • Heath (Moore) • Booth (Baguley) • Burns (Parrott) • Howard (Parrilon)
* **Lost 4-5 on penalties.** *Penalty-scorers:* Baguley • Burns • Howard • Parillon

TOURNAMENT SQUAD

Chris BAGULEY	Ian HOWARD
Ritchie BAKER	Michael LEA
Mitchell BOOTH	Kieron LEE
Aaron BURNS	James MOORE
Frazer CAMPBELL	Ashley PARILLON
Luke DANIELS	Chris PARROTT
Joe HEATH	Ryan SHAWCROSS
Sam HEWSON	Danny SIMPSON

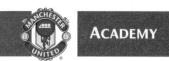

ACADEMY

SIXTH INTERNATIONAL FRIENDLY CHAMPIONSHIP OF SEVEN-A-SIDE FOOTBALL (UNDER 13s) – BARCELONA, SPAIN

Thursday 27 December 2001 **v PARIS ST GERMAIN (France) • Drawn: 1-1**

Ingram-Hughes • Chester • Kendrick • Cleverley • Drinkwater • Derbyshire • **Brandy**
Substitutes: Amos • Bryan • Eckersley • Rowe • Skidmore

Thursday 27 December 2001 **v REAL MADRID (Spain) • Lost: 1-5**

Ingram-Hughes • Chester • Kendrick • Cleverley • Drinkwater • Derbyshire • **Brandy**
Substitutes: Amos • Bryan • Eckersley • Rowe • Skidmore

Thursday 27 December 2001 **v VALENCIA (Spain) • Lost: 2-3**

Amos • Chester • Kendrick • Cleverley • Drinkwater • Derbyshire • **Brandy 2**
Substitutes: Bryan • Eckersley • Ingram-Hughes • Rowe • Skidmore

Friday 28 December 2001 **v ATHLETIC BILBAO (Spain) • Won: 2-1**

Amos • Eckersley • **Kendrick** • Derbyshire • Drinkwater • Bryan • **Brandy**
Substitutes: Chester • Cleverley • Ingram-Hughes • Rowe • Skidmore

TOURNAMENT SQUAD

Ben AMOS
Febian BRANDY
Antonio BRYAN
James CHESTER
Tom CLEVERLEY
James DERBYSHIRE

Daniel DRINKWATER
Richard ECKERSLEY
Dominic INGRAM-HUGHES
Matthew KENDRICK
Daniel ROWE
Alex SKIDMORE

TOURNOI SANS FRONTIERE
(UNDER 13s) 2002, SENS, FRANCE

v RENNES (France) Group C • Drawn: 1-1 — Friday 29 March 2002

Amos • Cleverley • Derbyshire • Kendrick • Chester • Drinkwater • Eckersley • Rowe • **Brandy** • Bryan • Mellor

v L'YONNE (France) Group C • Won: 4-0 — Saturday 30 March 2002

Amos • **Thompson** • Derbyshire • Crompton • Chester • **Coleman** • Eckersley • Butterfield • Brandy • **Hanson 2** • Mellor

Substitutes: Cleverley (Derbyshire) • Rowe (Brandy) • Bryan (Mellor)

v LILLE (France) Group C • Drawn: 0-0 — Saturday 30 March 2002

Amos • Thompson • Derbyshire • Kendrick • Chester • Drinkwater • Eckersley • Rowe • Brandy • Coleman • Mellor

Substitute: Bryan (Coleman)

v NANTES ATLANTIQUE (France) Second Stage • Lost: 0-1 — Saturday 30 March 2002

Amos • Cleverley • Derbyshire • Kendrick • Chester • Drinkwater • Eckersley • Rowe • Brandy • Bryan • Mellor

Substitute: Butterfield (Drinkwater)

v METZ (France) Second Stage • Lost: 0-3 — Sunday 31 March 2002

Amos • Cleverley • Derbyshire • Kendrick • Chester • Butterfield • Eckersley • Rowe • Brandy • Bryan • Mellor

v PARIS ST GERMAIN (France) Second Stage • Drawn: 1-1 — Sunday 31 March 2002

Amos • Thompson • Derbyshire • Kendrick • Chester • Drinkwater • Eckersley • Butterfield • Brandy • Hanson • Mellor

*Substitutes: **Bryan** (Thompson) • Crompton (Chester)*

v GENEVE (Switzerland) Seventh/Eighth Place Play-Off • Won: 2-1 — Sunday 31 March 2002

Amos • Cleverley • Derbyshire • Kendrick • Crompton • Drinkwater • Eckersley • Butterfield • **Brandy 2** • Bryan • Hanson

Substitutes: Chester (Kendrick) • Mellor

TOURNAMENT SQUAD

Ben AMOS	Theo COLEMAN	Matthew KENDRICK
Febian BRANDY	Jon CROMPTON	Thomas MELLOR
Antonio BRYAN	James DERBYSHIRE	Daniel ROWE
Jacob BUTTERFIELD	Daniel DRINKWATER	Joe THOMPSON
James CHESTER	Richard ECKERSLEY	
Tom CLEVERLEY	Lee HANSON	

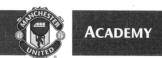

VZW MAARTEN CUP INTERNATIONAL YOUTH TOURNAMENT – BASSEVELDE, BELGIUM

Saturday 25 May 2002 v KUUKI BASSEVELDE (Belgium) Group A • Won: 5-0

Amos • Eckersley • Chester • Kendrick • Derbyshire • **Cleverley** • Thompson • Drinkwater • Mellor • **Brandy 3** • **Bryan**
Substitutes: Blackman • Butterfield • McGarvey • Skidmore • Wilkinson

Saturday 25 May 2002 v STANDARD LUIK (Belgium) Group A • Lost: 1-2

Amos • Eckersley • Chester • Kendrick • Derbyshire • Cleverley • **Thompson** • Butterfield • Mellor • Brandy • Bryan
Substitutes: Drinkwater • Blackman • McGarvey • Skidmore • Wilkinson

Saturday 25 May 2002 v RSC ANDERLECHT (Belgium) Group A • Lost: 0-4

Amos • Eckersley • Chester • Kendrick • Skidmore • Cleverley • Drinkwater • Derbyshire • Mellor • Blackman • Bryan
Substitutes: Brandy • Butterfield • Thompson • McGarvey • Wilkinson

Sunday 26 May 2002 v CLUB BRUGGE (Belgium) Play-Off • Drawn: 0-0*

Amos • Eckersley • Chester • Kendrick • Skidmore • Cleverley • Drinkwater • Derbyshire • Mellor • Blackman • Bryan
Substitutes: Brandy • Butterfield • Thompson • McGarvey • Wilkinson
* Lost 0-2 on penalties.

Sunday 26 May 2002 v STANDARD LUIK (Belgium) Seventh/Eighth Play-Off • Won: 3-0

Amos • Eckersley • Chester • Kendrick • Skidmore • Cleverley • Drinkwater • Derbyshire • **Mellor** • Blackman • Bryan
*Substitutes: **Brandy 2** • Butterfield • Thompson • McGarvey • Wilkinson*

TOURNAMENT SQUAD

Ben AMOS
Febian BRANDY
Nicky BLACKMAN
Antonio BRYAN
Jacob BUTTERFIELD
James CHESTER

Tom CLEVERLEY
James DERBYSHIRE
Danny DRINKWATER
Richard ECKERSLEY
Matt KENDRICK
Thomas MELLOR

Jay McGARVEY
Alex SKIDMORE
Joseph THOMPSON
Greg WILKINSON

OTHER EVENTS AT OLD TRAFFORD

PUBLIC TRAINING SESSION — Friday 10 August 2001

(Sir Alex Ferguson, Jimmy Ryan, Mike Phelan and the Manchester United First Team Squad)

Attendance: 6,388

FIFA WORLD CUP QUALIFIER – GROUP 9 — Saturday 6 October 2001

ENGLAND 2
Sheringham
Beckham

GREECE 2
Charisteas
Nikolaidis

Attendance: 66,090

RUGBY SUPER LEAGUE GRAND FINAL — Saturday 13 October 2001

BRADFORD BULLS 37
Tries: Withers 3
Lowes
Fielden
Mackay
Goals: Paul H. 5
Mackay
Drop Goal: Paul H.

WIGAN WARRIORS 6
Try: Lam
Goal: Furner

Attendance: 60,164

FRIENDLY INTERNATIONAL — Saturday 10 November 2001

ENGLAND 1
Beckham

SWEDEN 1
Mild

Attendance: 64,413

FA CUP (Sponsored by AXA) Semi-Final — Sunday 14 April 2002

MIDDLESBROUGH 0

ARSENAL 1
Festa o.g.

Attendance: 61,168

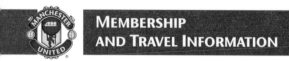

GENERAL INFORMATION

During the football season the Ticketing & Membership Services office hours are as follows:

Monday to Friday: 9.00am – 5.00pm
Home Match Days: 9.00am – kick-off

MEMBERSHIP

Once we deem Membership has reached its capacity, our books will close for the season and no further applications will be accepted. In the main, sales of match tickets for home games are restricted to members. It is therefore important to note that anyone wishing to attend a home game must become a member. Application forms are available upon request by telephoning **0870 442 1994**, to personal callers at the Ticketing & Membership Services office or by visiting our website at **www.manutd.com**

MEMBERS' PERSONAL ACCIDENT INSURANCE

Under our special personal accident insurance policy with Lloyds Underwriters, all members are insured whilst in attendance and travelling to and from the stadium (until safe return to current place of residence) for all competitive games played by the Manchester United 1st team, both home and away, anywhere in the world.

The following accidental death and bodily injury benefits apply:

1. Death £10,000 (limited to £1,000 for persons under 16 years of age)
2. Total and irrecoverable loss of sight of both eyes £10,000
3. Total and irrecoverable loss of sight in one eye £5,000
4. Loss of two limbs £10,000
5. Loss of one limb £5,000
6. Total and irrecoverable loss of sight in one eye and loss of one limb £10,000
7. Permanent total disablement (other than total loss of sight of one or both eyes or loss of limb) £10,000

The above is subject to the policy conditions and exclusions. Further details are available from the Membership Secretary to whom any enquiries should be addressed.

BRANCHES OF THE SUPPORTERS' CLUB

A full list of all our official branches of the supporters club can be found on pages 218 to 224.

AWAY TRAVEL

Domestic Games:

All Club Members, which includes Private Box holders, Executive Suite & Club Class Members and Season Ticket and League Match Ticket Book holders, are automatically enrolled in our Away Travel Club and, as such, are entitled to book coach travel from Old Trafford to all Premiership venues. Full details can be found on the opposite page.

How to make a Booking:

You can book a place on a coach, subject to availability, upon personal application at the Ticketing & Membership Services office, in which case you must quote your MUFC membership number. Alternatively, you can make a postal application by submitting the relevant payment, a stamped addressed envelope and a covering letter quoting your MUFC membership number. Telephone reservations are also acceptable during normal office hours on **0870 442 1994** if making payment by credit/debit card. Cancellations must be made in advance of the day of the game.

Car park attendants will be on duty should you wish to park your car on one of our car parks before travelling to an away game. This service is offered at no extra charge but we wish to point out that the Club will not be held responsible for any damage or theft from your vehicle.

Members are advised to check match ticket availability before booking a place on a coach. Details can be obtained by telephoning our Ticket & Match Information line on **0870 757 1968**.

MEMBERS' COACH TRAVEL FROM OLD TRAFFORD

Opponents	Executive Coach	Luxury Coach	*Departure Time	**Estimated Return Time to Old Trafford
Arsenal	£21.00	£16.00	8.30 am	9.30 pm
Aston Villa	£15.00	£11.00	11.30 am	7.30 pm
Birmingham City	£15.00	£11.00	11.30 am	7.30 pm
Blackburn Rovers	£11.00	£8.00	1.00 pm	6.15 pm
Bolton Wanderers	£11.00	£8.00	1.00 pm	6.15 pm
Charlton Athletic	£21.00	£16.00	8.00 am	10.00 pm
Chelsea	£21.00	£16.00	8.30 am	9.30 pm
Everton	£11.00	£8.00	1.00 pm	6.15 pm
Fulham	£21.00	£16.00	8.30 am	9.30 pm
Leeds United	£11.00	£8.00	1.00 pm	6.15 pm
Liverpool	£11.00	£8.00	1.00 pm	6.15 pm
Manchester City	NO CLUB TRAVEL AVAILABLE			
Middlesbrough	£16.00	£12.00	11.00 am	8.00 pm
Newcastle United	£17.00	£13.00	10.30 am	8.30 pm
Southampton	£21.00	£16.00	8.30 am	10.00 pm
Sunderland	£17.00	£13.00	10.30 am	8.30 pm
Tottenham Hotspur	£21.00	£16.00	8.30 am	9.30 pm
West Bromwich Albion	£15.00	£11.00	11.30 am	7.30 pm
West Ham United	£21.00	£16.00	8.30 am	9.30 pm
Millennium Stadium, Cardiff	£22.00	£17.00	7.00 am	11.00 pm

All times based on games with a 3.00 pm kick-off
* Departure times are subject to change and it is vital to check the actual time when making your booking
** Return times shown are only estimated and are subject to traffic congestion

EUROPEAN TRAVEL

The Ticketing & Membership Services office is also responsible for organising members travel and distribution of match tickets for our European away games. Full details will be made known when available, via all usual channels.

If you have any query or require further information regarding membership, domestic away travel, European away games, personal insurance or branches of the Supporters Club, please write to this address: Ticketing & Membership Services, Manchester United Football Club, Old Trafford, Manchester M16 0RA. Or, if you prefer, you can telephone the office on **0870 442 1994** or send a fax on **0161 868 8837**. R.N.I.D. Textphone **0161 868 8668**.

ABERDEEN Branch Secretary Michael Stewart, 15E Balnagask Road, Torry, Aberdeen AB11 8HU **Tel** 01224 890243 (home); **Mobile** 07740 980967. *Departure points* Guild Street, Aberdeen 6.00am; Forfar Bypass 6.45am; The Kingsway, Dundee 7.00am; Stirling Services 8.15am (coach for home games only). New members welcome – contact branch secretary for further information.

ABERGELE AND COAST Branch Secretary Eddie Williams, 14 Maes-y-Dre, Abergele, Clwyd, North Wales, LL22 7HW **Tel** 01745 823694. *Departure points* Aber; Llanfairfechen; Penmaen Mawr; Conwy; Llandudno Junction; Colwyn Bay; Abergele; Rhyl; Rhuddlan; Dyserth; Prestatyn; Mostyn; Holywell; Flint; Deeside.

ABERYSTWYTH AND DISTRICT Branch Secretary Alan Evans, 6 Tregerddan, Bow Street, Dyfed, SY24 5AW **Tel** 01970 828117 after 6pm. *Departure points* Please contact branch secretary.

ASHBOURNE Branch Secretary Diane O'Connell, 1 Milldale Court, Ashbourne, Derbyshire, DE6 1SN **Tel** 01335 346105 (evenings). *Departure points* The Maypole, Brook Street, Derby 11.30am (4.30pm); Markeaton Roundabout, Derby 11.45am (4.45pm); Hanover Hotel, Ashbourne 12 noon (5.00pm); Ashbourne Bus Station 12.05pm (5.05pm); (times in brackets denote 8.00pm evening fixtures). For 7.45pm fixtures depart 15 minutes earlier. Contact branch secretary for details of travel to away fixtures.

BARNSLEY Branch Secretary Mick Mitchell, 12 Saxon Crescent, Worsbrough, Barnsley, S70 5PY **Tel** 01226 283 983. *Departure points* Locke Park Working Mens Club, Park Road, Barnsley via A628 12.30pm (5.30pm) or 2½ hours before any other kick-off times.

BARROW AND FURNESS Branch Secretary Robert Bayliff, 183 Chapel Street, Dalton-in-Furness, Cumbria, LA15 8SL **Mobile** 07788 762936. *Departure points* Barrow, Ramsden Square 9.30am (4.00pm); Dalton 9.45am (4.15pm); Ulverston 10.00am (4.30pm) and A590 route to M6 (times in brackets denote evening fixtures).

BEDFORDSHIRE Branch Secretary Nigel Denton, 4 Abbey Road, Bedford, MK41 9LG **Tel** 0410 964329. *Departure points* Bedford Bus Station, pick-up at Milton Keynes 'Coachways', Junction 14, M1.

BERWICK-UPON-TWEED Branch Secretary Margaret Walker, 17 Lords Mount, Berwick-Upon-Tweed, Northumberland, TD15 1LY. Chairman Raymond Dixon, 92 Shielfield Terrace, Berwick-upon-Tweed **Tel** 01289 308671. SAE for all enquiries please. *Departure points* Berwick, Belford, Alnwick, Stannington, Washington; Scotch Corner, Leeming Bar and anywhere on the main A1 – by arrangement.

BIRMINGHAM Branch Secretary Paul Evans, 179 Longbridge Lane, Longbridge, Birmingham B31 4LA **Tel** 0121 604 1385 (6.30pm-9.00pm). Coaches operate to all home games. For times and additional information please telephone or send a stamped addressed envelope. *Departure points* Birmingham; Birmingham City Centre; Tennis Courts Public House (A34); Scott Arms and Junction 7 (M6).

BLACK COUNTRY The branch attend all home/away games. Coach details are as follows: *Departure points* St Lawrence Tavern, Darlaston 11.00am (4.00pm); Woden Public House, Wednesbury 11.10am (4.10pm); Friendly Lodge Hotel, J10, M6 11.15am (4.15pm); Wheatsheaf Public House, off J11, M6 11.25am (4.25pm) (times in brackets denote evening fixtures). For further information contact branch secretary Ade Steventon **Tel** 0121 531 0826 (6.30pm–9.00pm) **Mobile** 07931 714318 (6pm–9.30pm) or Ken Lawton **Tel** 01902 636393 (6.30pm–9pm).

BLACKPOOL, PRESTON AND FYLDE Chairman Martin Day **Tel** 01253 891301; **E-mail:** martin.day@endeavour.co.uk Travel Secretary Jean Halliday **Tel** 01772 635887. Coach pick-ups: Cleveleys, Bispham, 'Saddle', Blackpool, St Annes, Lytham, Preston. Social Secretary Tony Nicholson **Tel** 07760 226893 (we are always looking for friendly football matches).

BRADFORD AND LEEDS Branch Secretary Sally Hampshire, PO Box 87, Cleckheaton, West Yorkshire, BD19 6YN **Tel** 07973 904554. **Email:** ian.Hampshire@btinternet.com **www.bradfordreds.co.uk**

BRIDGNORTH AND DISTRICT Branch Secretary Ann Saxby, 30 Pitchford Road, Albrighton, Near Wolverhampton WV7 3LS **Tel** 01902 373260 *Departure points* Ludlow; Bridgnorth; Albrighton; Wolverhampton.

BRIDGWATER AND SOUTH WEST Branch Secretary Ray White, 4 Spencer Close, Bridgwater, Somerset, TA6 5SP **Tel** 01278 452186 **Mobile** 07850 950750 **E-mail:** raywhite@bridgwater-reds.co.uk **Website: www.bridgwater-reds.co.uk** *Departure points* Taunton; Bridgwater; Weston-super-Mare; Clevedon, Aztec West (Bristol).

BRIGHTON Branch Secretary Colin Singers, 34 Meadowview Road, Sompting, Lancing, West Sussex **Tel** 01903 761679 **Mobile** 07931 540723. *Departure points* Worthing Central 6.30am; Shoreham (George Pub) 6.40am; Brighton railway station 7.00am; Gatwick Airport 7.45am.

BRISTOL, BATH & DISTRICT Ticket Secretary Dennis Dunford, 26 Fontwell Drive, Downend, Bristol BS16 6RR **Mobile** 07989 586613 (6.00pm–8.00pm). Travel Secretary Julie Ladd, The Cart House, Poplar Farm, Stanton Prior, Bath, BA2 9HX **Mobile** 07759 733334 (6.00pm–8.00pm); Chairman Paul Biggs; Treasurer Eve Berry; Administrator Karen Pettinger; Committee Member Margaret Pettinger. *Departure points* Executive Coach 1: Keynsham Church; Bath Railway Station; Nailsworth; Sainsbury's Stroud; M5 Junction 13. Executive Coach 2: Bristol Temple Meads; Bradley Stoke North; M5 Junction 14.

BURTON-ON-TRENT Branch Secretary Mrs Pat Wright, 45 Foston Avenue, Burton-on-Trent, Staffordshire, DE13 0PL **Tel** 01283 532534. *Departure points* Moira (garage); Swadlincote; Burton (B&Q Lichfield Street); Stoke area.

CARLISLE AND DISTRICT Branch Secretary Arnold Heard, 28 Kentmere Grove, Morton Park, Carlisle, Cumbria, CA2 6JD **Tel/Fax** 01228 538262, **Mobile** 07860 782769. *Departure points* For departure times and details on the branch, please contact branch secretary.

CENTRAL POWYS Branch Secretary Bryn Thomas, 10 Well Lane, Bungalows, Llanidloes, Powys, SY18 6BA **Tel** 01686 412391 (home) 01686 413 200 (work). *Departure points* Crossgates 10.30am; Rhayader 10.45am; Llanidloes 11.05am; Newtown 11.25am.

CHEPSTOW AND DISTRICT Branch Secretary Anthony Parsons, 56 Treowen Road, Newbridge, Newport, Gwent, NP11 3DN **Tel** 01495 246253. *Departure points* Newbridge; Pontypool; Cwmbran Bus Station; Newport; Coldra Langstone; Magor; Caldicot; Chepstow. For departure times and further details contact branch secretary.

CHESTER AND NORTH WALES Branch Chairman Eddie Mansell, 45 Overlea Drive, Hawarden, Deeside, Flintshire, CH5 3HR **Tel** 01244 520332. Branch Secretary Mrs Kate Reynolds, 139 Park Avenue, Bryn-Y-Baal, Mold, Flintshire CH7 6TR **Tel** 01352 753962. Membership Secretary Mrs Irene Keidel, 3 Springfield Drive, Buckley, Flintshire CH7 2PH **Tel** 01244 550943. *Departure points* Oswestry; Ellesmere; Wrexham; Chester; Rhyl; Greenfield; Flint; Queensferry (ASDA store); Whitby (Woodlands); Ellesmere Port (bus station); Frodsham.

CLEVELAND Branch Secretary John Higgins, 41 Ashford Avenue, Acklam, Middlesbrough TS5 4QL **Tel** 01642 643112. Treasurer Brian Tose, 5 Cowbar Cottages, Staithes, Cleveland TS13 5DA **Tel** 01947 841628. *Departure points* Please contact branch secretary for details.

COLWYN BAY AND DISTRICT Branch Secretary Clive Allen, 62 Church Road, Rhos-on-Sea, Colwyn Bay, North Wales, LL28 4YS **Tel** 01492 546400. Branch Chairman Bill Griffith, 'Whitefield', 60 Church Road, Rhos-on-Sea, Colwyn Bay, North Wales, LL28 4YS **Tel** 01492 540240. *Departure points* bus stop Mostyn Broadway (opposite Asda stores) 11.00am (4.00pm); bus stop opposite Llandudno Junction railway station 11.15am (4.15pm); Guy's Newsagents, Conway Road, Colwyn Bay 11.30am (4.30pm); bus stop opposite Marine Hotel, Old Colwyn 11.35am (4.35pm); Top Shop, Abergele Road, Old Colwyn 11.40am (4.40pm); bus stop at Fair View Inn, Llandudlas 11.45am (4.45pm); Slaters Showrooms bus stop, Abergele 11.50am (4.50pm); Talardy Hotel, St. Asaph 12.00noon (5.00pm); Plough Hotel, Aston Hill, Queensferry 12.45pm (5.45pm) (times in brackets denote evening fixtures).

CORBY Branch Chairman Andy Hobbs, 32 Lower Pastures, Great Oakley, Corby, Northants **Tel** 01536 744 838 **Mobile** 07974 571353. Branch meetings 7.15pm first Sunday of the month, Lodge Park Sports Centre, Shetland Way, Corby. *Departure points* Co-op Extra Store, Alexandra Road, Corby 8.30am (1.30pm); Co-op Extra Superstore, Northfield Avenue, Kettering 8.40am (1.40pm) (times in brackets denote evening fixtures).

CRAWLEY Branch Secretary Jimmy Ahearne, 7 Greenwich Close, Broadfield, Crawley, West Sussex RH11 9LZ **Mobile** 0797 0334660.

CREWE AND NANTWICH Branch Secretary Andy Ridgway, 38 Murrayfield Drive, Willaston, Nantwich, Cheshire CW5 6QF **Tel** 01270 568418. *Departure points* Nantwich Barony 12.30pm (5.00pm); Earl of Crewe 12.40pm (5.10pm); Cross Keys 12.50pm (5.20pm) (times in brackets denote evening fixtures). Away travel subject to demand.

DONCASTER AND DISTRICT Branch Secretary Albert Thompson, 89 Anchorage Lane, Sprotboro, Doncaster, South Yorkshire, DN5 8EB **Tel** 01302 782964. Branch Treasurer Sue Moyles, 217 Warningtongue Lane, Cantley **Tel** 01302 530422 **Fax** 01302 349203 **Mobile** 07740 699824 **Email:** sfmoyles@hotmail.com Branch Chairman Paul Kelly, 58 Oak Grove, Conisbrough DN12 2HN **Tel** 01709 324058. Membership Secretary Mrs L Sudbury, 8 Parkway, Armthorpe, Doncaster **Tel** 01302 834323. *Departure points* Broadway Hotel, Dunscroft 10.30am (4.30pm); Edenthorpe 10.40am (4.40pm); Waterdale (opposite main library) 10.45am (4.45pm); The Highwayman, Woodlands 11.00am (5.00pm) (times in brackets denote 8.00pm kick-off). Meetings held first Monday of every month (unless there is a home match) in the Co-op Social Club (at the back of B&Q) at 7.30pm.

DORSET Branch Secretary Mark Pattison, 89 Parkstone Road, Poole, Dorset, BH15 2NZ **Tel** 01202 744348. *Departure points* Poole railway station 6.15am (10.30am); Banksome (Courts) 6.20am (10.35am); Bournemouth, 6.30am (10.45am); Christchurch (Bargates) 6.45am (11.00am); Ringwood 7.00am (11.15am); Rownham Services 7.15am (11.30am); Chieveley Services 8.30am (12.30pm) (times in brackets denote evening fixtures.

DUKINFIELD AND HYDE Branch Secretary Marilyn Chadderton, 12 Brownville Grove, Dukinfield, Cheshire, SK16 5AS **Tel** 0161 338 4892. *Departure points* Details of meetings and travel available from the above or S. Jones **Tel** 0161 343 5260.

EAST ANGLIA Branch Secretary Mark Donovan, 55 The Street, Holywell Row, Mildenhall, Bury St Edmonds, Suffolk IP28 8LT **Tel** 01638 717075 (9.00am–6.00pm) – details of your local representative can also be obtained by telephoning this number. Executive travel available to all home fixtures via the following services: Service No.1: Clacton; Colchester; Braintree; Great Dunmow; Bishop Stortford. Service No.2: Felixstowe; Nacton; Ipswich; Stowmarket; Bury St. Edmonds. Service No.3: Thetford; Mildenhall; Newmarket; Cambridge; Huntingdon. Service No.4: Lowestoft; Great Yarmouth; Norwich; East Dereham; Kings Lynn. Coaches also operate to all away games for which departure details are dependent on demand and ticket availability.

EAST MANCHESTER Branch Secretary Tony McAllister, 10 Walmer Street, Abbey Hey, Gorton, Manchester M18 8QP **Tel** 0161 230 7098 **Mobile** 07786 222596. Branch meetings held on the last Thursday of each month (8.00pm) at Gorton Labour Club, Ashkirk Street, Gorton, Manchester.

EAST YORKSHIRE Branch Secretary Ian Baxter, 18 Soberhill Drive, Holme Moor, York YO43 4BH **Mobile** 07768 821844. Hull Administrator Fred Helas **Mobile** 07774 775 078. *Departure points* Hull Coach: Hull Marina 10.30am (3.30pm). Howden Coach: Bay Horse, Market Weighton 10.30am (3.30pm); Redbrick Café, Howden; 11.00am (4.00pm) (times in brackets denote evening fixtures).

ECCLES Branch Secretary Gareth Morris, 11 Brentwood Drive, Monton, Eccles, Manchester, M30 9LP **Tel** 0161 281 9435. *Departure point* (away games only) Rock House Hotel, Peel Green Road, Peel Green, Eccles (for departure times please contact branch secretary).

FEATHERSTONE & DISTRICT Branch Secretary Paul Kingsbury, 11 Hardwick Road, Featherstone, Nr Pontefract, W Yorks WF7 5JA **Tel** 01977 793910 **Mobile** 07971 778161. Treasurer Andrew Dyson, 46 Northfield Drive, Pontefract, W Yorks WF8 2DL **Tel** 01977 709561 **Mobile** 07979 326183. *Departure points* Pontefract Sorting Office 11.30am (4.30pm); Corner Pocket, Featherstone 11.40am (4.40pm); Green Lane, Featherstone 11.45am (4.45pm); Castleford bus station 11.55am (4.55pm) (times in brackets denote evening fixtures). Meetings held every fortnight (Mondays) at the Jubilee Hotel, Wakefield Road, Featherstone.

FLEETWOOD Branch Secretary Stuart Gill, 24 Cleveleys Avenue, Cleveleys, Lancashire LA5 2AZ **Mobile** 07789 072390.

GLAMORGAN AND GWENT Branch Secretary Neil Chambers, 201 Malpas Road, Newport, South Wales NP20 5PP. Branch Chairman Cameron Erskine **Tel** 02920 623705 (10.00am–1.00pm Monday-Friday (answerphone at other times). Mobile 07885 615546 **E-mail:** c.erskine@ntlworld.co.uk *Departure points* Skewen; Port Talbot; Bridgend; Cardiff; Newport.

GLASGOW Branch Secretary David Sharkey, 45 Lavender Drive, Greenhills, East Kilbride G75 9JH **Tel** 01355 902592 (7–11pm). Coach run to all home games. *Departure points* Queen Street Station, Glasgow 8.00am (1.00pm); The Angel, Uddingston 8.15am (1.15pm); plus any M74 Service Stations (times in brackets denote evening fixtures).

GLOUCESTER AND CHELTENHAM Branch Secretary Paul Brown, 59 Katherine Close, Churchdown, Gloucester, GL3 1PB **Tel** 01452 859553 **Mobile** 07801 802593 **E-mail:** muscglos@aol.com *Departure points* Bennetts Yard, Eastern Ave, Glos. 8.45am (1.45pm); Station Road, Gloucester 9.00am (2.00pm); Cheltenham railway station (outside Midland Hotel) 9.10am (2.10pm); Cheltenham Gas Works Corner 9.15am (2.15pm) (times in brackets denote evening fixtures).

GRIMSBY AND DISTRICT Branch Secretary Bob England, 5 George Butler Close, Laceby, Grimsby, DN37 7WA **Tel** 01472 752130 **E-mail:** redbob68@hotmail.com Travel Arrangements Craig Collins (Branch Chairman) **Tel** 01472 314273. Membership Secretary Sarah Bell **Tel** 01472 314273.

GUERNSEY Branch Secretary Eddie Martel, Ayia Napa, Rue des Barras, Les Maresqets, Vale, Guernsey, Channel Isles **Tel** 01481 46285.

GWYNEDD Branch Secretary Gwyn Hughes, Sibrwd y Don, Tan y Cefn, Llanwnda, Caernarfon, Gwynedd, LL54 7YB **Tel** 01286 830073 **Mobile** 07050 380804 **E-mail** Gwyn.Hughes@manutd.com *Departure points* Pwllheli; Llanwnda; Caernarfon; Bangor (for departure times, please contact branch secretary).

HAMPSHIRE Branch Secretary Pete Boyd, 22 Weavers Crofts, Melksham Wilts SN12 8BP **Tel/Fax** 01225 700354 **E-mail** pete@muschants.com **Website:** www.muschants.com Membership Secretary/Treasurer: Roy Debenham, 11 Lindley Gardens, Alresford, Hampshire, SO24 9PU **Tel/Fax** 01962 734420. Chairman Paul Marsh, Oaktree Cottage, Commonhill Road, Braishfield, Hants. SO51 0QF **Tel** 01732 473570. *Departure points* (1) King George V playing fields, Northern Road, Cosham 7.30am (12.00 noon); (2) Sainsburys, Hedge End 7.50am (12.20pm); (3) Bullington Cross Inn, Junction of A34 & A303 8.20am (12.50pm); (4) Tot Hill Services (A34) just south of Newbury 8.40am (1.10pm).

HARROGATE AND DISTRICT Branch Secretary Michael Heaton, Railway Cottage, Grange Road, Dacre Banks, Harrogate, N Yorks HG3 4EF **Tel & Fax** 01423 780679 **Mobile** 07790 798328. *Departure points* include: Nidderdale; Rippon; Northallerton; Leyburn; Harrogate; Skipton and Earby areas. Coaches also operate to all away games, inc. European. For further information contact branch secretary. Send s.a.e for membership details. Meetings held every third Thursday in each month at the Hopper Lane Public House on the A59 leaving Harrogate.

HASTINGS Branch Secretary Tim Martin, 94 Gillsmans Hill, St Leonards-on-Sea, East Sussex TN38 0SL (NO PERSONAL CALLERS PLEASE) **Tel** 01424 442073 (6pm–8pm) **Mobile** 07973 656716 (daytime) **E-mail:** martin@silvan.fsnet.co.uk For match bookings phone Tim at the above. For Membership details and other enquiries, contact: Chris Fry **Tel** 01424 437595 **Mobile** 07973 309382; Steve Whitelaw **Tel** 07881 610345; Rod Beckingham **Tel** 01424 443477 (6pm–8pm) *Departure points* Eastbourne, Tesco's Roundabout 5.40am; Bexhill, Viking Chip Shop 6.00am; Silverhill Traffic lights 6.15am; Hurst Green, George Pub 6.40am; Pembury, Camden Arms Pub 7.00am (all above times for 3 or 4pm kick-off). For details of travel to away games please contact branch secretary.

HEREFORD Branch Secretary Norman Elliss, 40 Chichester Close, Abbeyfields, Belmont, Hereford, HR2 7YU **Tel** 01432 359923 **Fax** 01432 342880. *Departure points* Leominster 8.30am (2.00pm); Bulmers Car Park, Hereford 9.00am (2.30pm); Ledbury 9.30am (3.00pm);Malvern Link BP Garage 9.45am (3.15pm); Oak Apple Pub, Worcester 10.00am (3.30pm) (times in brackets denote mid-week fixtures).

HERTFORDSHIRE Organised travel to home and away games. Pick-up points at Hertford; Welwyn; Stevenage; Hitchin and Luton. Travel arrangements – contact Mick Prior **Tel** 01438 361900. Membership – contact Mick Slack **Tel** 01462 622451. Correspondence to: Steve Bocking, 64 Westmill Road, Hitchin, Herts. SG5 2SD **Tel** 01462 622076.

HEYWOOD Branch Secretary Denis Hall, 2 Hartford Avenue, Summit, Heywood, Lancs OL10 4XH **Tel** 01706 364475. Chairman Lee Swettenham, 30 Wilton Grove, Heywood, Lancs OL10 1AZ **Tel** 01706 368953. *Departure Point* Bay Horse, Torrington Street, Hopwood/Heywood 1.00pm (6.00pm midweek).

HIGHLANDS & ISLANDS Branch Secretary Kenneth MacAskill, 2 Claymore House, Croyard Road, Beauly, IV4 7DJ **Tel** 01463 783765 (6pm–10pm only).

HIGH PEAK Chairman Dave Rhodes, 21 Park Road, Whaley Bridge, High Peak SK23 7DJ **Tel** 01663 732484. Branch Secretary Keith Udale, 101 Station Road, Marple, Stockport SK6 6PA.

HYNDBURN & PENDLE Branch Secretary Alan Haslam, 97 Crabtree Avenue, Edgeside, Waterfoot, Rossendale, BB4 9TB **Tel** 01706 831736. *Departure points* Barnoldswick 11.15am (4.45pm); Nelson 11.30am (5.00pm); Burnley 11.45am (5.15pm); Accrington 12.15pm (5.45pm); Haslingden 12.20pm (5.50pm); Rawtenstall 12.30pm (6.00pm) (times in brackets denote evening fixtures).

INVICTA REDS (KENT) Branch Secretary Vic Hatherly **Tel** 01634 865613 **Mobile** 0773 668 6962. Tickets and Travel: Shaun Rogers or Louise Dodd **Tel** 01622 721344 (not after 9pm) **Mobile** 0781 388 0616 (not after 9pm). Correspondence to: Invicta Reds (Kent), Pop-In Newsagents, 97 Boundary Road, Ramsgate, Kent, CT11 7NP. **E-mail:** invictareds@manutd.com **Website:** www.invictareds.org.uk *Departure points* Pop-In Newsagents, Ramsgate; Mill Lane, Herne Bay; Magistrates Court, Canterbury; M2 Medway Services; M2, Junction 3, Chatham; Little Chef Services, A2 by Cobham; Dartford Tunnel; M25, Junction 28; M25, Junction 26.

ISLE OF MAN Branch Secretary Gill Keown, 5 King Williams Way, Castletown, Isle of Man, IM9 1DH **Tel** 01624 823143 **E-mail:** reddevil@manx.net

JERSEY Branch Secretary Mark Jones, 5 Rosemount Cottages, James Road, St. Saviour, Jersey, Channel Islands **Tel** 01534 34786 (home) 01534 885885 (work). Should any members be in Jersey during the football season, the branch shows television games in private club. Free food provided – everybody welcome, including children. Contact branch secretary for details.

KEIGHLEY Branch Secretary Kevin Granger, 3 Spring Terrace, Long Lee, Keighley, West Yorkshire, BD21 4SZ **Tel** 01535 661862 **Mobile** 01709 555653 **Fax** 01535 600554 **E-mail:** k.d.granger@talk21.com *Departure points* Coach leaves from Keighley Technical College in Cavendish Street then travels to Colne, and joins M65 & M66 to Manchester. Contact branch secretary for more details.

KNUTSFORD Branch Secretary John Butler, 4 Hollingford Place, Knutsford WA16 9DP **Tel** 01565 651360 **Fax** 01565 634792 **E-mail:** johnmbutler@onetel.net.uk Treasurer John Aston; Chairman Angus Campbell. Please contact the Secretary for details of meetings (usually weekly).

LANCASTER AND DISTRICT Branch Secretary Ed Currie, 30 Dorrington Road, Lancaster LA1 4TG **Tel** 01524 36797 **Mobile** 07880 550247. *Departure points* Carnforth Ex Servicemens 11.45am (4.45pm); Morecambe Shrimp Roundabout 12.00pm (5.00pm); Lancaster Dalton Square 12.20pm (5.20pm) then A6 route to Broughton Roundabout for M6 (times in brackets denote evening fixtures).

LEAMINGTON SPA Branch Secretary Mrs Norma Worton, 23 Cornhill Grove, Kenilworth, Warwickshire, CV8 2QP **Tel** 01926 859476 **E-mail:** norma.worton@virgin.net *Departure points* Newbold Terrace, Leamington Spa; Leyes Lane, Kenilworth; London Road, Coventry.

LINCOLN Branch Secretary Steve Stone, 154 Scorer Street, Lincoln, Lincolnshire, LN5 7SX **Tel** 01522 885671. *Departure points* Unity Square at 10.00am on Saturdays (3.00pm kick-off). Midweek matches, depart at 3.00pm from Unity Square.

LONDON Branch Secretary Ralph Mortimer, 55 Boyne Avenue, Hendon, London, NW4 2JL **Tel 0208 203 1213** (after 6.30pm).
Departure points Home Games - Coaches depart from following points: Semley Place, Victoria 8.00pm (12.30pm); Staples Corner 8.30am (1.15pm); Junction 11, (M1) 9.00am (1.45pm) (times in brackets denote evening fixtures).
A coach will run for every away game, depending on tickets. Please contact branch secretary after 6.30pm for details.

LONDON ASSOCIATION Branch Secretary Najib Armanazi **Tel 07941 124591** **E-mail: najcantona@hotmail.com** Membership Secretary Alison Watt **Tel 01322 558333** (7pm–9pm only) **E-mail: alisonwatt@redlodge.freeserve.co.uk**

LONDON FAN CLUB Branch Secretary Paul Molloy, 65 Corbylands Road, Sidcup, Kent, DA15 8JQ **Tel 0208 302 5826.** Travel Secretary Mike Dobbin.
E-mail: info@mulfc65.freeserve.co.uk
Departure points Euston Station by service train – meeting point at top of escalator from Tube. Cheap group travel to most home and away games.

MACCLESFIELD Branch Secretary Ian Evans, 25 Pickwick Road, Poynton, Cheshire SK12 1LD. Chairman Mark Roberts **Tel 01625 434362.** Treasurer Rick Holland, 97 Pierce Street, Macclesfield SK11 6EX **Tel 01625 427762.** Membership Secretary Neil McCleland **Tel 01625 613183.**
Departure points Home games, meet Macclesfield railway station 11.45am (4.45pm midweek fixtures). For away games, please contact branch secretary.

MANSFIELD Branch Secretary Peggy Conheeney, 48 West Bank Avenue, Mansfield, Nottinghamshire, NG19 7BP **Tel/Fax 01623 621140 Mobile 0776 1107104 E-mail: peg.con.musc@faxvia.net**
Departure points Kirkby Garage 10.00am (4.00pm); Northern Bridge, Sutton 10.10am (4.10pm); Mansfield Shoe Co. 10.20am (4.20pm); Pegs Home 10.30am (4.30pm); Young Vanish, Glapwell 10.40am (4.40pm); Hipper Street School, Chesterfield 10.55am (4.55pm) (times in brackets denote evening fixtures). Away games are dependent on ticket availability – please contact branch secretary.

MID-CHESHIRE Branch Secretary Leo Lastowecki, 5 Townfield Court, Barnton, Northwich, Cheshire, CW8 4UT **Tel 01606 784790.**
Departure points Please contact branch secretary.

MIDDLETON & DISTRICT Branch Secretary Kevin Booth, 8 Wicken Bank, Hopwood, OL10 2LW **Tel 0161 624196 Mobile 07762 741438.** Chairman Mike Conroy, 12 Lulworth Road, Middleton, Manchester 24 **Tel 0161 653 5696.**
Home Games: coaches depart Crown Inn, Middleton 1 hour prior to kick-off.
Away Games: contact branch secretary.

MILLOM AND DISTRICT Branch Secretary/Chairman Clive Carter, 47 Settle Street, Millom, Cumbria, LA18 5AR **Tel 01229 773565.** Treasurer Malcom French, 4 Willowside Park, Haverigg, Cumbria, LA18 4PT **Tel 01229 774850.** Assistant Treasurer Paul Knott, 80 Market Street, Millom, Cumbria **Tel 01229 772826.**

NEWTON-LE-WILLOWS Branch Chairman Mark Coleman, 14 Avocet Close, Newton-le-Willows **Tel 01925 222390.** Branch Secretary Mrs Joan Collins, Birley Street, Newton-le-Willows **Tel 01925 228959.** Ticket Secretary Anthony Hatch **Mobile 07909 580790.** Travel Secretary Mark Cheshire **Tel 01925 276298 Website: http/nlwmust.ukong.com** Meetings once a month in the Legh Arms public house, Newton-le-Willows. Telephone any of the above for date of meeting – all telephone enquiries before 9.00pm. Coach travel for selected home games to be booked and paid in advance. Most games available at Legh Arms. Junior and family membership welcome.

NORTH DEVON Branch Secretary Dave Rogan, Leys Cottage, Hilltop, Fremington, Nr Barnstaple, EX31 3BL **Tel/Fax 01271 328280 Mobile 07967 682167.**
Departure points Please contact branch secretary.

NORTH EAST Branch Secretary John Burgess, 10 Streatlam Close, Stainton, Barnard Castle, Co Durham, DL12 8RQ **Tel 01833 695200.**
Departure points Newcastle Central Station, 8.30am (1.00pm); A19/A690 roundabout 8.50am (1.20pm); Peterlee roundabout 9.00am (1.30pm); Hartlepool Baths 9.15am (1.45pm); Hartlepool Owton Lodge 9.20am (1.50pm); Hartlepool Sappers Corner 9.25am (1.55pm); Billingham, The Swan pub 9.30am (2.00pm); Darlington Feethams bus station 10.00am (2.30pm); Scotch Corner 10.10am (2.40pm); Leeming Bar Services A1 10.20am (2.50pm).

NORTH MANCHESTER Branch meetings at Leggatts Wine Bar, Oldham Road, Failsworth. Coaches to all home and away games. Secretary Graham May **Mobile 07931 505488.** All home coach details from Garry Chapman **Tel 07748 970225.** All away coach details from Dixie **Tel 07968 121872.** All other enquiries contact Graham **07931 505488.**

NORTH POWYS For all ticket and match enquiries and coach travel, contact Branch Secretary Glyn T Davies, 7 Tan-y-Mur, Montgomery, Powys, SY15 6PR **Tel 01686 668841.** Area Officials: Knighton – Mr R. Davies **01547 528318;** Welshpool – Mr Colin Harrington **01938 570571;** Newton – Mr P Owen **01686 610545** or Mr A.L. Jones **01686 610806.** Coaches leave: Saturdays: 8.30am for early kick-off; 10.30am for 3.00pm kick-off; midweek 4.00pm calling at Newtown, Abermule, Welshpool and Mile End Service Station, Oswestry. Branch Chairman: Mr B. Benyon **Tel 01691 670611.** Branch Treasurer Mrs B. Foulkes **Tel 01938 810979.** Branch meetings are held every eight weeks. For other enquiries telephone **01938 810979** or contact branch secretary.

NORTH STAFFORDSHIRE Branch Secretary Peter Hall, Cheddleton Heath House, Cheddleton Heath Road, Leek ST13 7DX **Tel 01538 360364.**
Departure points 12.30pm (5.15pm) Leek bus station (times in brackets denote evening fixtures).

NORTH YORKSHIRE Branch Secretary Andy Kirk, 80 Trafalgar Road, Scarborough, YO12 7QR **Tel/Fax 01723 372876 Mobile 07766 338164.**
E-mail andykirk25@yahoo.co.uk
Departure points Executive coaches to all home games from Whitby, Scarborough, Malton and York – booking in advance is required.
Please phone secretary for further details.

NOTTINGHAM Branch Secretary Wayne Roe, Vine Cottages, 15 Platt Street, Pinxton, Notts NG16 6NX **Tel 07870 604269** (home travel) **E-mail: wainy@aol.com** Martyn Meek **Tel 01773 768424** (away travel). *Departure points* Nottingham10.00am (3.00pm); Ilkeston 10.30am (3.30pm); Eastwood 10.45am (3.45pm); Junction 28, M111.00am (4.00pm) (times in brackets denote evening fixtures).

OLDHAM Branch Secretary Dave Cone, 67 Nelson Way, Washbrook, Chadderton, Lancashire, OL9 8NL **Tel 0161 626 9734 Mobile 07973 939255.** Chairman Martyn Lucas, 1 Wickentree Holt, Norden, Rochdale OL12 7PQ **Tel 01706 355728.** Meeting every Tuesday night 7.30pm–9.00pm at Horton Arms, 1 Ward Street, off Middleton Road, Chadderton, Oldham. Match Travel: coach to all home matches; Mid-week – leaves at 6.00pm; Weekend 3.00pm k.o. – leaves at 1.00pm; Weekend 4.00pm k.o. – leaves at 1.30pm. Away travel – subject to receiving match tickets.

OXFORD, BANBURY AND DISTRICT Branch Secretary Mick Thorne, "The Paddock", 111 Eynsham Road, Botley, Oxford OX2 9BY **Tel/Fax 01865 864924 E-mail: mickthorne@tinyworld.co.uk**
Departure points McLeans Coach Yard, Witney 8.00am (1.30pm); Botley Road Park-n-Ride, Oxford 8.30am (2.00pm); Plough Inn, Bicester 8.45am (2.15pm); bus station, Banbury 9.15am(2.30pm) (times in brackets denote evening fixtures). Mid-week European matches, coaches depart 30 minutes earlier.
Coach fare for home games: adults £12.00, Junior & OAPs £9.00. All coach seats must be pre-booked. Away travel, including European, subject to match tickets.

PETERBOROUGH AND DISTRICT Branch Secretary Andrew Dobney, 3 Northgate, West Pinchbeck, Spalding, Lincs, PE11 3TB **Tel 01775 640743 E-mail: andrew@dobney.fsnet.co.uk**
Departure points Spalding bus station 8.30am (1.15pm); Peterborough, Key Theatre 9.15am (2.00pm); Grantham, Foston Services 10.00am (2.45pm) (times in brackets denote evening fixtures).

PLYMOUTH Branch Secretary Dave Price, 34 Princess Avenue, Plymstock, Plymouth PL9 9EP **Tel 01752 482049.**
Departure Points Tamar Bridge 6.30am (10.30am); Bretonside 6.45am (10.45am); Plympton 7.00am (11.00am); Ivybridge 7.10am (11.10am); Buckfastleigh 7.25am (11.25am); Exeter Services 7.50am (11.50am) (times in brackets denote evening fixtures). Regular coach service to home games.

PONTYPRIDD Branch Secretary Lawrence Badman, 11 Laura Street, Treforest, Pontypridd, Mid Glamorgan, South Wales, CF37 1NW **Tel 01443 406894 Mobile 07855 621669 E-mail: lawrence@pmusc.fsnet.co.uk**
Departure points Treorchy, Porth; Pontypridd; Caerphilly and Newport. Membership Secretary: Paula Barry **Tel 01633 774223.** Away Travel Secretary Gareth Williams **Tel 01443 674505.** Phone calls to branch secretary between 5pm and 7pm only, answerphone at all other times.

REDDITCH Branch Secretary Mark Richardson, 90 Alcester Road, Hollywood, Worcestershire, B47 5NS **Tel/Fax 07890 584676.**
Departure points Redditch and Bromsgrove.

ROCHDALE Contact Paul Mulligan **01706 368909** for ticket/travel arrangements.

ROSSENDALE Branch Secretary Ian Boswell, 44 Cutler Lane, Stacksteads, Bacup, Lancs OL13 0HW **Tel 01706 874764 Mobile 07802 502356** (all enquiries).
Meetings: The Royal Hotel, Waterfoot – see local press or send e-mail to **ROYALREDS@theroyal-hotel.co.uk** Coach travel arrangements – contact Paul Stannard **01706 214493 (Fax) Tel 01706 215371 (Fax) or Paul@theroyal-hotel.co.uk**

RUGBY AND NUNEATON Branch Secretary Greg Pugh, 67 Fisher Avenue, Rugby, Warwickshire CV22 5HW **Tel 01788 567900.** Chairman Mick Moore, 143 Marston Lane, Attleborough, Nuneaton, Warwickshire **Tel 01203 343 868.** *Departure points* St Thomas Cross Pub, Rugby; McDonalds at Junction 2, M6, Coventry; Council House, Coton Road, Nuneaton. Departure times vary according to match.

RUNCORN AND WIDNES Branch Secretary Elizabeth Scott, 39 Park Road, Runcorn, Cheshire, WA7 4SS.

SCUNTHORPE Branch Secretary Pat Davies **Tel 01724 851359.** Chairman Guy Davies **Tel 01724 851359.** Transport Manager Tony Fish **Tel 01724 341029.**

SHEFFIELD & ROTHERHAM Branch Secretary Roger Everitt, 27 South Street, Kimberworth, Rotherham, South Yorkshire, S61 1ER **Tel 01709 563613.**
Coach Travel available to all home games. *Departure points* Saturdays: Rotherham (Nelle Denes) 11.00am; Sheffield (Midland Railway Station) 11.20am; Stockbridge 11.50am; Midweek games: Rotherham (Nelle Denes) 4.30pm; Meadowhall Coach Park 4.45pm. Kick-off times vary Sat/Sun – please contact branch secretary.

SHOEBURYNESS, SOUTH END AND DISTRICT Branch Secretary Bob Lambert, 23 Royal Oak Drive, Wickford, Essex, SS11 8NT **Tel 01268 560168.** Chairman Gary Black **Tel 01702 219072.**
Departure points Cambridge Hotel, Shoeburyness 7.00am; Bell public house, A127 7.15am; Rayleigh Weir 7.20am; McDonalds Burger Bar, A127 7.30a; Fortune of War public house, A127 7.40am; Brentwood High Street 8.00am; Little Chef, Brentwood By-pass 8.05am. Additional pick-ups by arrangement with branch secretary. All coach seats should be booked in advance. Ring for details of midweek fixtures.

SHREWSBURY Branch Secretary Martyn Hunt, 50 Whitehart, Reabrook, Shrewsbury, SY3 7TE **Tel 01743 350397.** Chirk Secretary Mike Davies **Tel 01691 778678.**
Departure points Reabrook Island; Abbey Church; Monkmoor Inn; Heathgates Island; Harlescott Inn; Hand Hotel, Chirk. Depart Reabrook at 10.30am for 3.00 & 4.00pm kick-off; depart Reabrook at 3.00pm for 7.30 & 8.00pm kick-off.

SOUTH ELMSALL & DISTRICT Branch Secretary Bill Fieldsend, 72 Cambridge St, Moorthorpe, South Elmsall, Pontefract, West Yorkshire, WF9 2AR **Tel 01977 648358 Mobile 07818 245954.** Treasurer Mark Bossons **Tel 01977 650316.** Meetings held every Tuesday at the South Kirkby Royal British Legion Club.
Departure points Cudworth Library 11.30am (4.30pm); Hemsworth Market 11.45am (4.45pm); Mill Lane 11.50am (4.50pm); Pretoria WMC 12 noon (5.00pm) (times in brackets denote evening fixtures).

SOUTHPORT Branch Secretary Mr B Budworth, 51 Dawlish Drive, Marshside, Southport **Tel 01704 211361.** Chairman Mr J. Mason, 57 Claremont Drive, Birkdale, Southport **Tel 01704 565466.** Treasurer Mr J.A. Johnson **E-mail: joseph.johnson1@btinternet.com** Membership Secretary Mr C. Rothwell, 37 Eamont Ave, Marshside, Southport **Tel 01704 213920.** Transport Secretary Mr R. Grimes, 19 Victory Ave, Blowick, Southport **Tel 01704 212439.**

STALYBRIDGE Branch Secretary Walt Petrenko **Mobile 07788 491977.** Chairman S. Hepburn **Tel 0161 344 2328.** Treasurer R.A. Wild **Tel 0161 338 7277.** Membership Secretary A. Baxter **Tel 01457 838 764.** Away travel Nigel Barrett **Mobile 0802 799482.** Home travel B. Wiliamson **Tel 0161 338 6832.**
Departure points branch is based at The Pineapple, 18 Kenworthy Street, Stalybridge. Landlord Addy Dearnaley **Tel 0161 338 2542.** Home coach leaves from The Pineapple 1½ hours before kick-off. Away coaches are arranged when applicable per game – coaches run most games.

STOKE-ON-TRENT Branch Secretary Geoff Boughey, 63 Shrewsbury Drive, Newcastle, Staffordshire ST5 7RQ **Tel/Fax 01782 561680** (home) **Mobile 07768 561680 E-mail: geoff.boughey@btinternet.com**
Departure points Hanley bus station 12.00noon (5.00pm); School Street, Newcastle 12.10pm (5.10pm); Little Chef A34 12.15pm (5.15pm); The Millstone pub, Butt Lane 12.30pm (5.30pm) (times in brackets denote evening fixtures).
Branch meetings every Monday night. Contact branch secretary for details.

STOURBRIDGE & KIDDERMINSTER Branch Secretary Robert Banks, 7 Croftwood Road, Wollescote, Stourbridge, West Midlands DY9 7EU **Tel 01384 826636.**
Departure Points Contact branch secretary for departure points and times.

SURREY Branch Membership Secretary Mrs Maureen Asker, 80 Cheam Road, Ewell, Surrey, KT17 1QF **Tel 0208 393 4763.** Home League Games Co-ordinator John Ramsden, 22 Pound Lane, Godalming, Surrey **Tel 01483 420909.** Cup Games Co-ordinator John Fuggle, Flat 9, The Shrubbery, 22 Hook Road, Surbiton, Surrey **Mobile 07703 650869.**

SWANSEA Branch Secretary Dave Squibb, 156 Cecil Street, Mansleton, Swansea, SA5 8QJ **Tel 01792 641981 E-mail: david.squibb@manutd.com**
Departure points Swansea (via Heads of Valleys Road); Neath; Hirwaun; Merthyr; Tredegar; Ebbw Vale; Brynmawr; Abergavenny; Monmouth.

SWINDON Branch Secretary Martin Rendle, 19 Cornfield Road, Devizes, Wiltshire, SN10 3BA **Tel 01380 728358** (between 8.00pm and 10.00pm Monday to Friday).
Departure point Kingsdown Inn, Stratton St Margaret, Swindon.

SWINTON Branch Secretary John Berry, 20 Castleway, Clifton, Swinton, M27 8HX **Mobile 07887 676811**

TELFORD Branch Secretary Sal Laher, 4 Hollyoak Grove, Lakeside, Priorslee, Telford, TF2 9GE **Tel 01952 299224.**
Departure points Saturday (3pm kick-off) Cuckoo Oak, Madeley 10.30am; Heath Hill, Dawley 10.40am; Bucks Head, Wellington 10.50am; Oakengates 11.00am; Bridge, Donnington 11.10am; Newport 11.20am. Midweek (8.00pm kick-off) departure starts 4.30pm with ten minutes later for each of the above locations. Contact branch secretary for membership and further details.

TORBAY Branch Secretary Vernon Savage, 5 Courtland Road, Shiphay, Torquay, Devon TQ2 6JU **Tel 01803 616139 Fax 01803 616139 Mobile 07765 394238.**
Departure points Upper Cockington Lane, Torquay 7.00am; Newton Abbot railway station 7.20am; Kingsteignton Fountain 7.30am; Countess Wear Roundabout, Exeter 7.45am; Taunton 8.15am. Other departure times by arrangement with branch secretary. Midweek coach departure times – add 5 hours to above times.

UTTOXETER & DISTRICT Branch Secretary Mrs T A Bloor, 63 Carter Street, Uttoxeter, Staffordshire ST14 8EY. Branch Chairman Mr R Phillips, 77 Bentley Road, Uttoxeter **Tel 01889 567323.** Travel to matches leaving Smithfield Hotel, Uttoxeter 11.30am Saturday, and 4.30pm for night games.

WALSALL Branch Secretary Ian Robottom, 157 Somerfield Road, Bloxwich, Walsall WS3 2EN **Tel 01922 861746.**
Departure points Junction 9 (M6) 10.50am (4.15pm); Bell pub, Bloxwich 11.15am (4.50pm); Roman Way Hotel, A5 Cannock 11.30am (5.15pm); Dovecote Pub, Stone Road, Stafford 11.50am (5.35pm).

WARRINGTON Branch Secretary Su Buckley, 4 Vaudrey Drive, Woolston, Warrington, Cheshire, WA1 4HG **Tel 01925 816966.**
Departure points Blackburn Arms 1.00pm (6.00pm); Churchills 1.10pm (6.10pm); Chevvies 1.15pm (6.15pm); Highway Man/Kingsway 1.20pm (6.20pm); Rope 'n' Anchor 1.25pm (6.25pm) (times in brackets denote evening fixtures).

WELLINGBOROUGH Branch Secretary Phil Walpole, 7 Cowgill Close, Cherry Lodge, Northampton NN3 8PB **Tel/Fax 01604 787612.**
Departure points Shoe Factory, Irchester Road, Rushden 8.30am (1.30pm); Doc Martins Shoe Factory, Irchester 8.35am (1.35pm); The Cuckoo public house, Woolaston 8.45am (1.45pm); Police station, Wellingborough 8.55am (1.55pm); Duke of York public house, Wellingborough 9.00am (2.00pm); Trumpet public house, Northampton 9.10am (2.10pm); Abington Park bus stop, Northampton 9.15 am (2.15pm); Campbell Square, Northampton 9.20am (2.20pm); Mill Lane Layby (opposite Cock Hotel public house), Kingsthorpe 9.25am (2.25pm); Top of Bants Lane (opposite Timken), Dugton 9.30am (2.30pm).

WEST CUMBRIA Branch Secretary Robert Wilson, 23 Calder Drive, Moorclose, Workington, Cumbria CA14 3NZ **Tel 01900 872804 Mobile 07786 542607 E-mail: rob_in_the_trafford@hotmail.com**
Departure points Coach 1: Egremont 9.45am (3.15pm): Cleator Moor 10am (3.30pm); Whitehaven 10.15am (3.45pm); Distington 10.20am (3.50pm); Cockermouth 10.35am (4.05pm). Coach 2: Salterbeck 9.45am (1.45pm); Harrington Road 9.50am (1.50pm); Workington 10am (2.00pm); Station Inn 10.10am (2.10pm); Netherhall Cr 10.12am (2.12pm); Netherton 10.15am (2.15pm); Dearham 10.20am (2.20pm) (times in brackets denotes 8pm kick-off) – contact branch secretary for other kick-off times.

WEST DEVON Branch Secretary Mrs R.M. Bolt, 16 Moorview, North Tawton, Devon, EX20 2HW **Tel 01837 82682** (all enquiries).
Departure points North Tawton; Crediton; Exeter.

WESTMORLAND Branch Secretary Dennis Alderson, 71 Calder Drive, Kendal, Cumbria, LA9 6LR **Tel 01539 728248 Mobile 0973 965373.**
Departure points Ambleside; Windermere; Staveley, Kendal and Forton Services. For departure times and further details, please contact branch secretary.

WORKSOP Branch Secretary Mick Askew, 20 Park Street, Worksop, Nottinghamshire **Tel 01909 486194.**

YEOVIL Branch Secretary Richard Chapman-Cox, 34 Crofton Avenue, Yeovil, Somerset BA21 4DL **Tel 01935 478285 Mobile 07930 505349 E-mail: richard.chapmancox@btinternet.com**
Departure points Yeovil and Taunton. Transport available to non-branch members. Please contact branch secretary for departure times.

MANCHESTER UNITED DISABLED SUPPORTERS' ASSOCIATION – (MUDSA) Branch Secretary Phil Downs, M.U.D.S.A., PO Box 141, South D.O., M20 5BA **Tel 0161 434 1989 Fax 0161 445 5221 E-mail: phil.downs@cwcom.net**

IRISH BRANCHES

ABBEYFEALE & DISTRICT Branch Secretary Denis O'Sullivan **Tel 068 32525** or **086 8157146.** Chairman Denis Daly **Tel 068 31712** or **087 9880015.** Vice Chairman Gerard Foley **Tel 068 41725748.** Treasurer Paddy Finucane **Tel 068 32036.** Youth Officer Richard O'Mahony **Tel 068 32305** or **087 2055031.** Public Relations Officer Tomas Mann **Tel 068 31025** or **087 9130180.**
Regular meetings held at Donal and Ann's Bar, Abbeyfeale – contact branch secretary for more details.

ANTRIM TOWN Branch Secretary Brendan O'Neill, 86 Ballycraigy Road, Glengormley, Co Antrim BT36 4SX **Tel 028 90 842929.** Chairman William Cameron, 92 Donegore Drive, Parkhall, Antrim, N Ireland **Tel 02894 461634.** Club meetings held every other Thursday in the 'Top of the Town Bar', Antrim. All members must be registered with Manchester United's official membership scheme.

ARKLOW & SOUTH LEINSTER Branch Secretary James Cullen, 52 South Green, Arklow, Co Wicklow, Eire **Tel 087 2327859** or **0402 39816.**
All trips arranged via local committee members. Pick-ups Waterford to Dublin. Anyone interested in joining, please contact the Secretary.

BALLYCASTLE Branch Secretary Miss Cathy McLaughlin, 29 Caman Park, Ballycastle, Co Antrim, Northern Ireland BT54 6LW **Tel 028 207 68639.**

BALLYMONEY Branch Secretary Malachy McAleese, 8 Riverview Park, Ballymoney, Co Antrim, Northern Ireland BT53 7QS **Tel 028 276 67623.** Chairman Gerry McAleese, 11 Greenville Avenue, Ballymoney, Co Antrim, Northern Ireland **Tel 028 276 65446.**
Departure point Ballymoney United Social Club, Grove Road, Ballymena; Belfast Harbour or Belfast International Airport. Meetings: Last Thursday of every month, Ballymoney United Social Club, 35 Castle Street, Ballymoney **Tel 028 276 66054** – New members always welcome. **Website: www.musc-ballymoney.co.uk E-mail: info@musc-ballymoney.co.uk**

BANBRIDGE Branch Secretary James Loney, 83 McGreavy Park, Derrymacash, Lurgan, Northern Ireland BT66 6LR **Tel 028 38 345058 Mobile 07901 833076.** Chairman Kevin Nelson, 10 Ballynamoney Park, Derrymacash, Lurgan, N Ireland **Tel 028 38 344232 Mobile 07879 436358.**
Departure Points Corner House, Derrymacash; Lurgan Town Centre; Newry Road, Banbridge.

BANGOR Branch Secretary Gary Wilsdon, 4 Bexley Road, Bangor, Co Down, BT19 7TS **Tel 028 91 458485 E-mail: gary.wilsdon@virgin.net** Branch meetings held every other Monday 8.00pm at the Imperial Bar, Central Avenue, Bangor.

BELFAST REDS Branch Secretary John Bond, 53 Hillhead Crescent, Belfast, Northern Ireland, BT11 9FS **Tel 028 90 627861.**

BUNDORAN Branch Secretary Danny Tighe, "United Cottage", The Rock, Bundoran, Co Donegal, Eire **Tel & Fax 072 42080 Mobile 086 859 7718.**
Departure point The Holyrood Hotel and additional pick-up points en route to Dublin Port. All bookings to be made through branch secretary only. Bookings should be made well in advance as travel arrangements have to be made. New members are welcome.

CARLINGFORD LOUTH Branch Secretary Harry Harold, Mountain Park, Carlingford, Co Louth, Ireland **Tel 00 353 42 9373379.**

CARLOW Branch Secretary Michael Lawlor, Trafford House, 20 New Oak Estate, Carlow, Ireland **Tel 0503 43759 Mobile 086 8950030** (Mon–Friday 7.00pm–9.00pm only). Treasurer William Carroll **Mobile 086 8593062** (Mon–Fri 9.00am–5.00pm only).

CARRICKFERGUS Branch Secretary Gary Callaghan, 3 Red Fort Park, Carrickfergus, Co Antrim, Northern Ireland BT38 9EW **Tel 028 93 355362 Fax 028 93 369995 E-mail: aca@globalnet.co.uk**
The branch holds their meetings fortnightly on a Monday evening at 8.00pm in the Quality Hotel, Carrickfergus. New members are welcome, especially Family and Juniors. The branch presently has a membership of 165 and organises trips to Old Trafford for all home games. They also travel to away matches including European whenever possible.

CARRYDUFF Branch Secretary John White, 'Stretford End', 4 Baronscourt Glen, Carryduff, Co Down, Northern Ireland, BT8 8RF **Tel & Fax 028 90 812377 E-mail: whitedevil@btopenworld.com** Chairman John Dempsey, 16 Baronscourt Glen, Carryduff BT8 8RF **Tel/Fax 028 90 812823 E-mail: john.dempsey@btinternet.com** Vice-Chairman Wilson Steele **Tel 028 94 464987.**
Branch website: www.musc-carryduff-branch.co.uk
Departure points The branch organise coach trips to Old Trafford for every home game from The Royal Ascot, Carryduff and The Grand Opera House, Belfast. Branch meetings are held every week. No alcohol and no other club colours are permitted on the coach. New members, particularly juniors, are always welcome as the branch has a strong family and cross community ethos. Branch membership exceeds 400 and ALL members must be registered with Manchester United's Official Membership Scheme. The branch owns a number of season tickets, which are used on trips.

CASTLEDAWSON Branch Secretary Niall Wright, 22 Park View, Castledawson, Co Londonderry, Northern Ireland **Tel 028 79 468779.**

CASTLEPOLLARD Branch Secretary Anne Foley, Coole, Mullingar, Co Westmeath, Ireland **Tel/Fax 00 353 44 61613 E-mail: muscpollard@hotmail.com**
Departure points The Square, Castlepollard. Additional pick-up points by arrangement with branch secretary. Branch meetings on third Monday of every month. Notification of additional meetings by newsletter.

CASTLEWELLAN Branch Secretary Seamus Owens, 18 Mourne Gardens, Dublin Road, Castlewellan, Co Down, Northern Ireland, BN31 9BY **Tel 028 437 78137 Fax 028 437 70764 Mobile 07714 756 455.** Chairman Tony Corr **Tel 028 437 22885** Treasurer Michael Burns **Tel 028 437 78665.**

CITY OF DERRY Branch Secretary David Kee, 35 Curlew Way, Waterside, Londonderry BT47 6LQ **Tel 028 71 34 4059 E-mail: secretary@codmusc.org.uk** Meetings on first Tuesday of every month at the Upstairs Downstairs Bar, Dungiven Road, Londonderry at 8.30pm.

CLARA Branch Secretary: Michael Kenny, River Street, Clara, Co Offaly, Ireland.

CLONMEL Branch Secretary Anthony O'Sullivan, No. 41 Honeyvine Estate, Clonmel, Co. Tipperary, Ireland.

COLERAINE Branch Secretary Noel Adair, 106 Lisnablaugh Road, Harper's Hill, Coleraine, Co Derry, Northern Ireland **Tel 028 703 57744.**

COMBER Branch Secretary Derek Hume, 14 Carnesure Hts., Comber, Co Down **Tel (028) 91 872608.** Chairman Stephen Irvine Branch **E-mail Comberbranch@onetel.net.uk**
Branch meetings are held on various Tuesdays. Details of these meetings are printed in 'The Newtownards Chronicle' newspaper and also available to view on our website www.propertysnaps.co.uk/CD.

COOKSTOWN Branch Secretary Geoffrey Wilson, 10 Cookstown Road, Moneymore, Co Londonderry, Northern Ireland BT45 7QF **Tel 028 86748625 Mobile 07855 760981 E-mail: gwilson@telco4u.net**
Meeting: First Monday of every month at above address – 9.00pm. New members are welcome however, all members must be registered with Manchester United's official membership scheme.

CORK AREA Branch Secretary Paul Kearney, Beech Road, Passage West, Co Cork, Republic of Ireland **Tel 021 841190.**

COUNTY CAVAN Chairman Owen Farrelly **Tel 046 42184** Secretary Gerry Heery **Tel 087 6181295.** Assistant Secretary Jimmy Murray **Tel 086 8289504 E-mail co.cavanbranch@eircom.net Website: www.cocavanbranch.homestead.com** Meetings on third Monday of each month in Tyrrells, Main St, Mullagh, Co Cavan.

COUNTY LONGFORD Branch Secretary Seamus Gill, 17 Springlawn, Longford, Republic of Ireland **Tel 043 47848 Fax 043 41655** Chairman Harry Ryan, 58 Teffia Park, Longford, Co. Longford. Treasurer Nicola King, 18 Harbour Row, Longford, Co Longford. President George Wenman.

COUNTY MONAGHAN Chairman Peter O'Reilly. Branch Secretary Seamus Gallagher. Assistant Secretary John Hughes. Treasurers Ann Devine & Jane Flynn. Meetings fortnightly throughout the season at Bellevue Tavern, Dublin Street, Monaghan. Secretary phone nos. **047 83265/81577 (home)** or **0868 307689 E-mail: seamusgallagh16@hotmail.com**

COUNTY ROSCOMMON Branch Secretary Noel Scally, Cashel, Boyle, Co Roscommon, Ireland **Tel 079 64995 Mobile 087 2228466.** Chairman Seamus Sweeney, Croghan, Boyle, Co Roscommon **Tel 079 68061 Mobile 087 6484931.** Treasurer Ray Livingstone, Shankill, Elphin, Co Roscommon **Mobile 087 6771230.** Meetings are held on third Thursday of every month at the Royal Hotel, Boyle, Co Roscommon.

COUNTY TIPPERARY Branch Secretary Mrs Kathleen Hogan, 45 Canon Hayes Park, Tipperary, Republic of Ireland **Tel 062 51042.**

COUNTY WATERFORD Branch Secretary Kevin Moore, 92 Childers Estate, Dungarvan, Co Waterford **Tel 086 3925677.** Chairman Oliver Drummy, 8 Cloneety Terrace, Dungarvan, Co Waterford. Vice-Chairman Tommy Keating, Ringnasillogue, Childers Estate, Dungarvan, Co Waterford. Treasurer Judy Connors, Hillview Drive, Dungarvan, Co Waterford. There are committee meetings held at least once a month and general meetings whenever necessary. Anyone in the Waterford region feel free contact the secretary for membership details and how to join.

CRAIGAVON Branch Secretary Eamon Atkinson, 8 Rowan Park, Tullygally Road, Craigavon, Co Armagh, Northern Ireland BT65 5AY **Tel 028 38 343870.** Chairperson Noel Flynn, 2 Avondale Manor, Craigavon **Tel 028 38 327788** Treasurer Susan Atkinson, 8 Rowan Park, Craigavon BT65 5AY **Tel: 028 38 343870.**
Departure Points Lurgan; Craigavon; Portadown; Tandragee; Dundalk; Dublin Port; Meetings held first Tuesday of each month at the Goodyear Sports & Social Club, Silverwood, Craigavon.

DONEGAL Branch Secretary Liam Friel **Tel (00 353) 87 6736967.** Chairman Paul Dolan. Treasurer Paddy Delap. Travel Organiser Tony Murray. Public Relations Officer W. Diver.

DOWNPATRICK Branch Secretary Terry Holland, 20 Racecourse Road, Downpatrick, Co Down, Northern Ireland **Tel/Fax 028 44 616467 Mobile 07712 622242.**

DUNDALK Chairman Michael McCourt. Secretary Arthur Carron. Treasurer Mary Laverty. Ticket & Travel Dickie O'Hanrahan. Committee members Ollie Kelly, Gery Dullaghan.

DUNGANNON Branch Secretary Ian Hall, 'Silveridge', 229 Killyman Road, Dungannon, Co Tyrone, Northern Ireland BT71 6RS **Tel 028 87 723085 (home) Tel 028 87 752255 (work) Mobile 07787 124765.**
Meetings every two weeks (all year) at 30 Church Street, Dungannon. For details on membership, meetings, and trips contact branch secretary or Keith Houston on **028 87 722735** or Lawrence McKinley **07867 941163.**

EAST BELFAST Branch Secretary John Dickson, 6 Martin Street, Belfast, BT5 4HG.

ENNIS Branch Secretary Seamus Hughes, 'Old Trafford', Quin, Ennis, Co Clare, Republic of Ireland **Tel 065 68 20282 Mobile 086 239 3975.** Branch Chairman Eamon Murphy, Knockboy, Ballynacally, Co Clare, Ireland **Tel 065 68 28105.** Meetings held at Roslevan Arms, Tulla Road, Ennis.

FERMANAGH Branch Secretary Gabriel Maguire, 80 Glenwood Gardens, Enniskillen, BT74 5LT **Tel 028 66 325 950 Mobile 07788 421739.** Chairman Eric Brown, 166 Main Street, Lisnaskea. Treasurer Raymond McBrien, Ardlougher Road, Irvinestown. Meetings held in Charlie's Lounge, Enniskillen.

FIRST BALLYCLARE Branch Secretary Alan Munce, 7 Merion Park, Ballyclare, Co Antrim, Northern Ireland, BT39 9XD **Tel 028 93 324126.**

FIRST NORTH DOWN (BANGOR) Branch Secretary Robert Quee, 'Stretford End', 67 Springhill Road, Bangor West, Co Down, Northern Ireland, BT20 3PD. Chairman: Walter Geary, 25 Beaumont Drive, Bangor BT19 6WH. First North Down supporters meet on alternative Tuesday evening at 8.00pm at Ballykillaire Sports Complex, Old Belfast Road, Bangor. New members always welcome. Branch operates a 'Family Package Membership'. For further details please ring the Secretary **Tel 028 91 453094 Mobile 07790 761828** or the Chairman **Tel 028 91 462732 Mobile 07803 109429.**

FIRST PORTAFERRY Branch Secretary David Peacock, 5 Loughshore Road, Portaferry, Northern Ireland, BT22 1PD. **Tel 028 427 28420/28646 Fax 028 427 29834.** Chair Tony Cleary. Treasurer Hugh Conlon. Branch meetings held first Tuesday every month @ 9.00pm at McNamara's, High Street, Portaferry.

FOYLE Branch Secretary Martin Harkin, 2 Harvest Meadows, Dunlade Road, Greysteel, Co Derry, Northern Ireland BT47 3BG. *Departure point* Ulsterbus Club, Bishop Street, Derry City. Travel Arrangements: meet Ulsterbus at midnight, boat at 2.50am on matchday. Hotel Comfort Friendly, Hyde Road. Return boat 2.30pm, arrive Ulsterbus Club 8.30pm.

GALWAY Branch Secretary Patsy Devlin, 97 Renville Village, Oranmore, Galway, Ireland **Tel 00 353 091 790929 Fax 00 353 87 2530366.**
(1) Meetings held monthly in Currans Hotel, Eyre Square. (2) All live TV games at Brennans Bar, New Docks. (3) Membership open all year round.

GLENOWEN Branch Secretary Jim Turner, 4 Dermot Hill Drive, Belfast, Northern Ireland BT12 7GG **Tel 02890 242682 Mobile 07990 848 961** (day)
E-mail: Jimmy.Turner@tesco.net

IVEAGH YOUTH Branch Secretary Russell Allen, 2 Iveagh Crescent, Belfast, Northern Ireland, BT12 6AW **Tel 028 90 542651 (office) 028 90 329621 (home).** Assistant Branch Secretary Brendan McBride, 3 Gransha Park, Belfast BT11 8AT **Tel 028 90 522400 (work), 028 90 203171 (home).**

IRELAND (DUBLIN) Branch Secretary Eddie Gibbons, 19 Cherry Orchard Crescent, Ballyfermont, Dublin 10 **Tel 01 626 9759 Fax 01 6236388**
Email: **muscirlbranch@hotmail.com.** Membership Secretary Michael O'Toole, 49 Briarwood Lawn, Mulmuddart, Dublin 15 **Tel 01 821 5702.**

KILKENNY Branch Secretary John Joe Ryan **Tel 056 6565827** (day) **056 65136** (after 6pm) **Fax 056 64043.** Branch Chairman Pat Murray **Tel 056 71772.**

KILLALOE & ROSCREA Branch Secretary Michael Flynn, 611 Cross Roads, Killaloe, Co Clare, Ireland **Tel 061 376031.** Chairman Seamus Doran, 7 Limerick Street, Roscrea **Tel 0505 23194.**

KILLARNEY Branch Secretary Frank Roberts, St Margaret's Road, Killarney, Co Kerry, Republic of Ireland. Chairman Bill Keefe. Treasurer Denis Spillane. Meetings held on the first Wednesday of every month at which future trips are organised.

LAGAN Branch Secretary John Mooreland, 29 Ashgrove Road, Newtownabbey, Co Antrim, BT36 6LJ.

LAOIS Branch Secretary Denis Moran, Newpark, Portlaoise, Co Laois, Ireland **Tel 0502 22681.**

LARNE Branch Secretary Brian Haveron, 69 Croft Manor, Ballygally, Larne, Co Antrim BT40 2RU **Tel 028 28 261197** (day) **028 28 583027** (night) **Mobile 07785 388959.** Branch Chairman John Hylands, 43 Olderfleet Road, Larne, Co Antrim BT40 1AS **Tel 028 28 277888.** Meetings: Every Monday night 8.00pm at St. John's Social Club, Mill Brae, Larne. The branch has an allocation for every home fixture and is a family orientated branch. New members always welcome.

LIMAVADY Branch Secretary Gerry Cooke, 20 Whitehill Park, Limavady, Co. Derry BT49 0QE **Tel 028 77 768080** (after 6pm) **Mobile 07903 236108.**

LIMERICK Branch Secretary Dennis O'Sullivan, 14 Rossa Avenue, Mulgrave Street, Limerick, Republic of Ireland **Tel 061 311502 Mobile 086 8435828.**

LISBURN Branch Secretary Colin Scott, 7 Barban Hill, Dromore, Co Down, Northern Ireland, BT25 1PR **Tel 028 92 699608 Mobile 07808 532951**
E-mail: **lisburnmusc@gcs-internet.com** The branch meets each Tuesday night at 8.30pm at the Club Rooms on Sackville Street. To join the branch you must be an official member of Manchester United. The branch travel to all games – league and European – and some away. Anyone interested in joining – families and kids welcome – please contact the branch secretary.

LISTOWEL Branch Secretary Aiden O'Connor, 55 Pytha Fold Road, Withington, Manchester M20 4UR **Tel 0161 434 4713.** Assistant Secretary David O'Brien, Bedford, Listowel, Co Kerry Ireland **Tel 068 22250.**

LURGAN Branch Secretary John Furphy, 123 Drumbeg North, Craigavon, Co Armagh, Northern Ireland BT65 5AE **Tel 028 38 341842.**

MAYO Branch Secretary Seamus Moran, Belclare, Westport, Co Mayo, Ireland **Tel 00 353 982 7533 (home) 00 353 985 5202 Mobile 00 353 872 417966 Fax 00 353 982 8874.** Chairperson Liam Connell, 70 Knockaphunta, Castlebar, Co Mayo, Ireland. Treasurer T J Gannon, 4 The Paddock, Castlebar Road, Westport, Co Mayo, Ireland. PRO: Kieran Mongey, Blackfort, Castlebar, Co Mayo, Ireland.

MEATH Branch Secretary Colm McManus, 46 Beechlawn, Kells, Co Meath, Republic of Ireland **Tel 046 49831.** *Departure points* for travel to Old Trafford: Jack's Railway Bar, Kells; Fairgreen; Naven.

NEWRY Branch Secretary Brendan McConville, 14 Willow Grove, Newry, Co Down, Northern Ireland, BT34 1JH **Tel 028 3026 6996**
E-mail: brendan.mcconville@manutd.com Chairman Jeffrey Clements **Tel 028 3026 7158.** Meetings held on first Tuesday of each month at the Cue Club, Newry **Tel 028 3026 6066.**

NEWTOWNARDS Branch Secretary Leo Cafolla **Tel 07710 820300 Fax 028 91 822200.** Chairperson Mrs Ruth Quann. A family orientated club who meet once a fortnight at Nixx Sport's Bar, Newtownards. New members always welcome.

NORTH BELFAST Branch Secretary Robert Savage, 47 Mayfield Road, Newtownabbey, Northern Ireland BT36 7WD **Tel 028 90 847237.** Meetings are no longer held at the Shamrock Social Club, please contact branch secretary if you require additional information.

OMAGH Branch Secretary Brendan McLaughlin, 4 Pinefield Court, Killyclougher, Omagh, Co Tyrone, Northern Ireland BT79 7YT **Tel 028 82 250025 Mobile 077 10 366 486.**

PORTADOWN Branch Secretary Harold Beck, 23 Kernan Grove, Portadown, Co Armagh, BT63 5RX **Tel 028 3 833 6877 Mobile 07703 360423.**

PORTAVOGIE Branch Secretary Robert McMaster, 6 New Road, Portavogie, Co Down BT22 1EN.

PORTRUSH Branch Secretary James Friel, 15-17 Causway Street, Portrush, Northern Ireland.

PORTSTEWART Branch Secretary Ryan McLaughlin **Tel 028 777 50281** (home) **Mobile 07764 533 446 E-mail: ryan.mclaughlin2@btopenworld.com** Club meetings held every second Wednesday of the month at Edgewater Hotel, Portstewart.

ROSTREVOR Branch Chairman John Parr, 16 Drumreagh Park, Rostrevor BT34 3DU **Tel 028 417 39797.** Branch Secretary Roger Morgan, 23 Ardfield Crescent, Warrenpoint, Co Down, Northern Ireland **Tel 028 417 54783.** Treasurer John Franklin, 14 Rosswood Park, Rostrevor, Co Down BT34 3DZ **Tel 028 417 38906.** Assistant Secretary M. Rea, 8 The Square, Rostrevor, Co. Down **Tel 028 417 39808.** Club President Paul Braham.

SION MILLS Branch Secretary Jim Hunter, 122 Melmount, Sion Mills, Co Tyrone, Northern Ireland, BT82 9EU **Tel 028816 58226 (home) 02882 252491 (work).**

SLIGO Branch Chairman Eddie Gray, 27 Cartron Heights, Sligo, Republic of Ireland **Tel 00 353 71 44387 Mobile 086 6075 855.** Branch Secretary Martin Feeney, 40 Cartron Bay, Sligo, Republic of Ireland. **Mobile 087 2971842.**

SOUTH BELFAST Branch Secretary James Copeland, 17 Oakhurst Avenue, Blacks Road, Belfast BT10 0PD **Tel 028 90 615184 or 028 90 871231 Mobile 07767 271648.** Chairman Danny Nolan. Vice-Chairman Michael Murphy. Treasurer James McLaughlin. Fundraising Officer Simon Murray.
Departure Point Balmoral Hotel, Blacks Road.

STEWARTSTOWN Branch Secretary Stephen Coyle, 8 Coolnafranky Park, Cookstown, Co Tyrone, Northern Ireland BT80 8PN **Tel 028 86 765511.**

STRABANE Branch Secretary Gerry Donnelly, 27 Dublin Road, Strabane, Co Tyrone, Northern Ireland, BT82 9EA **Tel 02871 883376.**

TALLAGHT Branch Secretary Jimmy Pluck, 32 Kilcarrig Cresent, Fettercairn, Tallaght, Co Dublin 24, Republic of Ireland **Tel/Fax 00 353 1 2442413 (home) Mobile 086 8030123** (anytime).

TIPPERARY TOWN Branch Secretary John Ryan, 19 Lakeland's, Tipperary Town, Co Tipperary, Republic of Ireland **Tel 00 353 86 883 1456 Fax 00 353 62 82059.**

TOWER ARDS Branch Secretary Stephen Rowley **Tel 028 91 810457 (home) 028 90 432014 (office).** Meetings held ever second Sunday in the Tower Inn, Mill Street, Newtownards.

TRALEE Branch Secretary Johnny Switzer, Dromtacker, Tralee, Co Kerry, Republic of Ireland **Tel 066 7124787.**

WARRENPOINT Branch Secretary Pat Treanor, 31 Oakland Grove, Warrenpoint **Tel 028 417 73921 Mobile 07775 968595.** Chairman John Bird, 23 Greendale Crescent, Rostrevor, Co Down **Tel 028 417 3837.** Treasurer Leo Tohill, 46 Carmen Park, Warrenpoint, Co Down **Tel 028 417 72453.** Club website address: **www.muwp/manutd.htm.** Club based at Cearnogs Bar, The Square, Warrenpoint, Co Down, N Ireland **Tel 028 417 53429.**
Branch meets last Friday of every month at 8.00pm.

WEST BELFAST Branch Secretary John McAllister, 25 Broadway, Belfast BT12 6AS **Tel 028 90 329423 Fax 0870 0637348 E-mail hoyt@lineone.net**
Branch Chairman George McCabe, 21 Beechmount Street, Belfast, BT12 7NG. Treasurer Mr G. Burns. Committee Mr Liam Curran, Mr Mark Mallon, Mr Michael Curran. Meetings held fortnightly on Tuesday evening in the 'Red Devil Bar', Falls Road, Belfast. For information contact branch secretary.

OVERSEAS BRANCHES

BELGIUM Chairman Peter Bauwens, Grote Markt 78/2, 9060 Zelzate, Belgium. **Tel 00 32 934 20403 Fax 00 32 934 20406.** Branch Secretary Kristof Haes, John Schenkelstraat 3, 9060 Zelzate, Belgium. **Tel 00 32 934 56474.**

CANADA Manchester United Supporters Club, 12 St Clair Avenue East, PO Box 69057, Toronto, Ontario, M4T 3AI, Canada. Chairman Kevin Kerr. For membership information **E-mail: chairman@muscc.com Website: www.muscc.com Fax 00 1 416 480 0501** fao Maureen.

CYPRUS Branch President Ronis Soteriades, P.O.Box 51365, 3504 Limassol, Cyprus **Tel 00 357 25337690 Fax 00 357 25388652.**

GERMAN FRIENDS Branch President Marco Hornfeck, Silberstein 36, 95179 Geroldsgrün, Germany **Tel 09267 8111**

GERMAN KREFELD REDS Branch Secretary Andy Marsh, Innsbrucker Str, 47807 Krefeld, Germany **Tel/Fax 00 49 (0) 2151 392908 Mobile 00 49 (0) 173 250 3390 E-mail: AndrewM63@aol.com** Assistant Branch Secretary Stuart Dykes, Grete Schmitz Str. 8, 47829 Kreffeld, Germany **Tel 00 49 (0) 2151 435 167 Fax 00 49 2151 435 168 Mobile 00 49 (0) 172 398 5152 E-mail: stuart.dykes@t-online.de** John McFadyen, Wisseler Str 13, 47574 Gcoh, Germany **Tel 00 49 (0) 2823 928504. Mobile 00 49 (0) 173 5203 933 E-mail: john.mcfadyen@mantud.com**

GERMAN REDS Branch Chairman Markus Nerlich, Eissendorfer Str 28, D-21073 Hamburg, Germany **Tel 00 49 40 76 75 32 02 Fax 00 49 40 30 01 41 11 E-mail: markusnerlich@aol.com**

GIBRALTAR Branch President C.A. Moberley; Branch Secretary D.R. Peralta. Treasurer B. Cardona; Membership Secretary Wilfred Gavito. Committee Members: R. Beiso, W. Lima, M. Ferro. Manchester United Supporters Gibraltar Branch, PO Box 22, Gibraltar **Tel (00 350) 76846/77475 Fax (00 350) 71608.**

HOLLAND Branch Secretary Ron Snellen, PO Box 33742, 2503 BA Den Haag, Holland **Tel 00 31 70 329 8602 Fax 00 31 70 367 2247 Internet: www.dutch-mancunians.nl E-mail: dennisvandervin@hetnet.nl**

HONG KONG 12B Shun Ho Tower, 24-30 Ice House Street, Central, Hong Kong **Tel 00 852 2869 1993 Fax 00 852 2869 4312.** Branch Secretary/Treasurer Rick Adkinson. Chairman Mark Saunders **E-mail: muschkb@pacific.net.hk**

ICELAND Branch Secretary Bubbi Avesson, Studningsmannaklubbur, Manchester United á Íslandi, PO Box 12170, 132 Reykjavik, Iceland.

LUXEMBOURG Branch Secretary Steve Kaiser **Tel 00 352 4301 33073 (work) 00 352 340265 (home).**

MALTA Quarries Square, Msida MSD 03, Malta (since 1959). **Tel 00 356 223531 Fax 00 356 231902 E-mail: musc@maltanet.net.mt Website: www.maltazone.com/hosted/mufc** Branch Secretary: Joseph Tedesco. Branch President Franco Mizzi

MAURITIUS Branch Secretary Yacoob Atchia, Flamingo Pool House, Remeno Street, Rose Hill, Mauritius, Indian Ocean **Tel 464 7382/454 7761/454 3570/464 7750 Fax 454 7839 E-mail: abyss.manutd@intnet.mu** Chairman Swallay Banhoo **Tel 464 4450 (home)** Treasurer Naniel Baichoo Tel 454 3570 (work) 465 0387 (home).

NEW SOUTH WALES Chairperson Steve Griffiths. Vice-Chairperson Tony Redman. Treasurer Jeanette Frost. Secretary John Panaretto. Founders Fred & Ann Pollitt. Branch Address P.O.Box 693, Sutherland, New South Wales 1499, Australia **Tel/Fax 00 61 2 982 29781 Website: manutd-nsw.one.net.au/index.htm**

NEW ZEALAND Branch Chairman Brian Wood, 55 Pine Street, Mount Eden, Auckland, New Zealand. Secretary Gillian Goodinson, 20 Sandown Road, Rothesay Bay, Auckland, New Zealand **E-mail: woody.utd@xtra.co.nz**

SCANDANAVIAN Branch Secretary Per H. Larsen, PO Box 4003 Dreggen, N-5835 Bergan, Norway **Tel +47 5530 2770** (Mon–Fri 08.00–16.00) **Fax +47 5596 2033 E-mail: muscsb@united.no**

SOUTH AFRICA PO Box 2540, Capetown 8000, S Africa **Tel 00 27 82 231 64364** (Customer care) **Fax 00 27 21 438 8295 E-mail: m.united@mweb.co.za**

SOUTH EAST ASIA Manager Jeremy Goon, 6-B Orange Grove Road, Singapore 258332 **Tel 00 65 737 0677 Fax 00 65 733 5073 E-mail: members@manutd-sea.com.sg**

SOUTH AUSTRALIA PO Box 276, Ingle Farm, South Australia 5098 **Fax 08 82816731.** Branch Secretary Mick Griffiths **Tel 08 82644499.** Branch Chairman Chris Golder **Tel 08 82630602.** Vice-Chairman John Harrison **Tel 08 82603413.** Treasurer Charlie Kelly **Tel 08 82628245.** Meetings are held at the Para Hills Soccer Club, Bridge Road, Para Hills, SA. The Manchester United Supporters Amateur League Soccer team train and play at Para Hills Soccer Club.

SWISS DEVILS Branch Secretary Marc Tanner, Dorfstrasse 30d, 5430 Wettingen, Switzerland **Tel (00 41 56) 426 94 80 Website: www.swissdevils.ch E-mail: vonisan@yahoo.co.uk**

TOKYO Branch Secretary Hiroki Miyaji, 2-24-10 Minami-Ayoma, Minato-ku, Tokyo, Japan **Tel +81 3 3470 3441** English Information Stephen Ryan **Tel +81 3 3380 8441 E-mail: best-oz@kk.iij4u.or.jp**

USA MUSC USA Branch HQ, PO Box 4199, Huntington, NY 11743, USA **Tel 00 1 631 547 5500** (day) **Fax 00 1 631 547 6800** (day) **Tel/Fax 00 1 631 261 7314** (evening) **E-mail: muscusa@muscusa.com Website: www.muscusa.com** General Secretary Peter Holland. Membership Secretary Trevor Griffiths Daytime **Tel 00 1 718 381 5300 (Ext 23) E-mail: tgmufc@aol.com**

MUSCUSA WEST COAST Membership Secretary Siamak Emadi, 26321 Eva St, Laguna Hills, CA 92656-3108 **Tel 00 1 949 661 2660 Ext. 127** (day) **E-mail: Siamak@taa.com**

VICTORIA, AUSTRALIA President Kieran Dunleavy **Tel/Fax (03) 9 850 8109.** Postal Address Manchester United Supporters Club of Victoria, PO Box 1199, Camberwell, 3124 Victoria **Website: www.vicmanutd.com E-mail: muscovic@vicnet.net.au**

WESTERN AUSTRALIA Branch Chairman Graham Wyche, 19 Frobisher Avenue, Sorrento 6020, Perth, Western Australia **Tel/Fax (08) 9 447 1144 Mobile 0417 903 101 E-mail: freobook@omen.com.au**